Adenomyosis:

A Significantly Neglected and Misunderstood Uterine Disorder

Maria Yeager

Copyright© 2016 All rights reserved. No part of this publication may be reproduced or transmitted in any form or be any means, electronic or mechanical, including photocopying, recording, or by any information storage and retrieval system, without the written permission of the author and except where permitted by law.

ISBN-13: 978-1533065117
ISBN-10: 153306511X

Cover design by Heidi Sutherlin, www.mycreativepursuits.com

Important notices:
Many of the supplements in this book have not been evaluated by the U.S. Food and Drug Administration. The supplements and statements in this book are not intended to diagnose, treat, cure or prevent adenomyosis or any other disease. The author accepts no responsibility for any illness or harm as a result of the use or misuse of the supplements described in this book.

The recommendations in this book are based on the author's own research of clinical studies. The author is not a physician. This book is not intended as a substitute for the medical advice of physicians. The reader should regularly consult a physician in matters relating to his/her health and particularly with respect to any symptoms that may require diagnosis or medical attention.

Although the author and publisher have made every effort to ensure that the information in this book was correct at press time, the author and publisher do not assume and hereby disclaim any liability to any party for any loss, damage, or disruption caused by errors or omissions, whether such errors or omissions result from negligence, accident, or any other cause.

Table of Contents

Preface 7
For a Moment, Imagine the Pain 11
Chapter 1 - What is Adenomyosis? 13
Chapter 2 - History of Adenomyosis and Endometriosis 19
Chapter 3 - Anatomy and Function of the Uterus 23
Chapter 4 - Symptoms of Adenomyosis 29
Chapter 5 - What are the Risk Factors? 33
Chapter 6 - So What Goes Wrong? 37
Chapter 7 - So What is Estrogen Dominance? 43
Chapter 8 - How Is Adenomyosis Diagnosed? 49
Chapter 9 - Junctional Zone Abnormalities 55
Chapter 10 - How is Adenomyosis Treated? 59
Chapter 11 - Infertility and Adenomyosis 69
Chapter 12 - Could Diet Play a Role? 73
Chapter 13 - Liver Detoxification 83
Chapter 14 - All About Xenoestrogens 89
Chapter 15 - Can Phytoestrogens Help? 101
Chapter 16 - Supplement Review and Recommendations for Adenomyosis 107
Chapter 17 - Omega-3 Fatty Acids May Offer Some Hope 119
Chapter 18 - We Desperately Need More Research! 125
Abbreviations 135
Definitions 137
References 147

Preface

Adenomyosis…this uterine disorder is not only difficult to deal with physically, but it is also a bear to research! I decided to take on this long and difficult process because I struggled for seventeen years with this disorder, and I can deeply empathize with anyone who is currently dealing with it. Not only is it a horribly painful disorder, but it is also a significantly neglected one by the medical and scientific community.

My story began at the age of fourteen with my first menstrual period. I had terrible cramps from day one. During my teenage years, I suffered from extremely heavy bleeding, anemia, and intensely painful cramps. I was told that this was "normal" and that some women just had it worse than others. So, with my ibuprofen and maxi pads in hand, I would go to school and put up with the pain and inconveniences of being a woman.

At the age of 25, I had the first of many attacks of debilitating pain. I was at the end of my period. I woke up in the middle of the night to excruciating pain in my lower abdomen, and I could barely walk to the bathroom. Waves of pain came about every three to four minutes, and each time a cramp hit me, I became faint and nauseated. The waves of pain began in my lower abdomen and moved into my back and down to the upper parts of my legs. It felt like a vice grip on my entire lower abdomen. I have never had children, but if I didn't know any better, I could swear I gave birth.

My mom drove to my apartment to take me to the hospital. When she arrived, I barely made it to the door to open it. I told her that there was no way I could walk to the car. With gently coaxing from her, I did make it to the car even though I was doubled over from the pain. Holding my belly and unable to stand up straight, I entered the hospital hoping that the wait wouldn't be long since I didn't know how long I could stand the pain. Suddenly, I had a terrible wave of pain and the urge to have a bowel movement. I rushed to the bathroom and had a terrible bout of diarrhea. Thankfully, when I came out of the bathroom, the nurse called us back to the emergency room.

After examining me, the ER physician told me that he thought I had food poisoning. Since I was in so much pain, the nurse gave me a shot of narcotic pain medication. After that, I don't remember much as I slept most of the next day. When I finally woke up, the pain was gone, and I was thankful that it was over.

About a year passed without any more attacks of excruciating abdominal pain, but I did continue to have extremely heavy periods, pre-menstrual migraines, severe menstrual cramps, and anemia. In general, during my menstrual periods, I felt like I had been hit by a truck. Each month, I was in severe pain for several days. I always wondered why I was so weak that I couldn't put up with my period discomforts. After all, other girls around me seemed to breeze right through their periods. What was wrong with me?

Then the nightmare began…full force. I woke up again to excruciating waves of abdominal pain. Sweat poured down my face as once again, that vice grip had taken hold of my lower abdomen. I held onto the bathroom sink as I became faint and saw stars. Knowing that I was about to faint, I tried to control my breathing and position myself where I wouldn't hit my head if I fell. I became more and more nauseated as the cramps continued, and eventually, I vomited due to the pain. As this horrendous night continued, I felt like I needed to have a bowel movement. I tried, but I was unable to defecate. I couldn't understand why I was having such a problem, and I pushed as hard as I could, but the constipation was relentless. After several hours, I eventually did have a bowel movement, but it was once again diarrhea. After this, the pain slowly let up, but I was exhausted and spent the next several days in bed as I recovered.

These attacks became more and more frequent with similar symptoms each time. Eventually I was able to predict when they would happen as my lower abdomen would bloat up right before an attack. I would sometimes look three to four months pregnant. I knew something was terribly wrong, but I was unable to get any help from the medical profession. They were unable to diagnose my condition properly. At one point, I was diagnosed with irritable bowel syndrome (IBS), and, as I found out later, that diagnosis was incorrect.

Over the years that I dealt with adenomyosis, I visited a slew of physicians, took more prescription medications than I can count, had more pap smears than any woman should have in her lifetime, had my thyroid tested dozens of times (each time it was normal), and had multiple surgeries. A laparoscopy was able to identify endometriosis, and it was removed through laser cauterization; however, the pain came back two months later. A hysterosonogram identified a uterine polyp, and it was removed through hysteroscopy. The pain continued. I had several D&Cs (dilation and curettage) for heavy bleeding which also helped for several months, but the problem always returned. Finally, in 2007, I had an endometrial ablation, and it failed. I began to bleed just twenty-four hours after surgery. My doctor finally agreed with me that it was time to consider hysterectomy.

The hysterectomy was performed about a month later. The uterine tissue was sent to a pathology lab where they confirmed that I had been suffering from severe diffuse adenomyosis with possible fibroids. Once the uterus was removed, all of my symptoms subsided. I never again had an attack of excruciating abdominal pain like I had when my uterus was still intact.

In addition to all of my painful physical symptoms, I also had to deal with the emotional aspect of this disorder. I was unable to get pregnant, and I have no children. Also, because the doctors could not find the cause of my pain, some people automatically assumed that I was making it all up. It is because of this physical and emotional pain that I am writing this book. My goal is to educate both the general public and the medical community on the severity of this disorder and the incredibly negative impact it can have on the quality of the lives of women who suffer from it. It is also imperative that additional research be done on adenomyosis as very little is known about it. Even though some progress has been made recently, much more needs to be done.

For women who suffer from adenomyosis, I hope you find this book useful in dealing with your symptoms. For the medical community, I hope this book propels you to refer patients with these symptoms to experts in the field of adenomyosis and excision surgery. For the scientific community, I implore you to continue research into the cause of adenomyosis and to find more effective ways to diagnose this neglected uterine condition.

For a Moment, Imagine the Pain

I wrote the following blog in 2015, and the response was overwhelming. In fact, the post went viral. I share it here to give the reader an inside look at what it is actually like to live with adenomyosis.

For the next few minutes, I ask you to put yourself in another person's shoes. Just imagine.

Imagine waking up in the middle of the night to excruciating pain that comes in waves, first in your lower abdomen and then moving to your lower back. These waves of pain come every three to four minutes, and are similar to full stage labor pains or kidney stone pain.

Imagine not knowing the reason or cause of this pain.

Imagine that you have no way to control this pain. The doctors have given you all kinds of medications, but nothing works.

Imagine going through this pain for five to six hours during an attack...waves of intense pain every three to four minutes which then start to move down to the upper parts of your legs. You could swear you are giving birth.

Imagine standing at the bathroom sink in the middle of all this with sweat pouring off your face and horrible nausea due to the terrible waves of pain. You can't stand up straight because the pain is so unbearable.

Imagine holding onto the sides of the bathroom sink as you try not to faint as yet another wave of pain hits you. You see stars, and you try to position yourself so that you won't hit your head if you fall.

Imagine an intense wave of pain throughout your belly as you grab onto the toilet to vomit...multiple times.

Imagine lying on the bathroom floor in the fetal position as you cry out of frustration while you are forced to endure this nightmare.

Imagine having menstrual periods that last ten to fourteen days per month with spotting on the other days.

Imagine having so much blood loss that you soak a pad in an hour.

Imagine how tired you feel because of the chronic anemia.

Imagine that you pass blood clots that are as big as the palm of your hand.

Imagine that you have so much abdominal bloating that you look three to four months pregnant.

Now imagine that this happens to you at least once a month.

Imagine trying to get pregnant while enduring all of this, but it never happens. You never have children.

Imagine the anxiety that you feel because you never know when an attack will hit you. You make sure you are always close to a bathroom. You panic as you drive down the highway and start to feel pelvic pain.

Imagine going through this while trying to hold a full-time job. What will your boss or co-workers say when you take another sick day?

Imagine trying to be a parent while suffering from this uterine condition. You can't take a sick day as a parent.

Imagine that you undergo numerous invasive tests only to be told that they can't find the cause of your problems.

Imagine being told that you need to see a psychologist because of this problem, and you are put on antidepressant medication for your depression and anxiety.

Imagine your friends, acquaintances, and "experts" telling you that "it's all in your head" because the doctors can't find a cause of the pain.

Imagine going through multiple surgeries but the pain and heavy bleeding always return.

Imagine having an endometrial ablation and being told that this will certainly stop the bleeding. The bleeding returns twenty-four hours after surgery.

Imagine having a hysterectomy before finally obtaining a correct diagnosis...after years of unbearable physical, mental and emotional pain. It was adenomyosis.

Imagine a doctor telling you that he doesn't know anything about adenomyosis. He tells you to "google it".

Just imagine. Imagine the frustration. Imagine the pain. Imagine your quality of life during that time.

Imagine...

Chapter 1 - What is Adenomyosis?

Adenomyosis is a uterine disorder that can cause a whole host of problems including painful and prolonged menstruation, heavy bleeding, and an enlarged uterus. A comprehensive list of all the symptoms can be found in Chapter 4. It can dramatically reduce the quality of a woman's life because of the excruciating pain, fatigue, anemia from excessive blood loss, and the emotional pain associated with fertility problems, just to name a few. It has been noted to be an estrogen-dependent disease (Yamanaka et al., 2014).

In Chapter 3, we will get into a more detailed discussion of the female reproductive tract. For now, to explain it in simple terms, the uterus has two main layers – the endometrium and the myometrium. The endometrium is the inner layer and is shed each month in the form of a menstrual period. The myometrium is the outer uterine muscle that contracts during childbirth and menstruation. In a normal uterus, these layers are distinct and separate. However, in adenomyosis, for unknown reasons, the endometrium invades the myometrium. During menstruation, these endometrial implants within the myometrium respond to hormonal stimulation, and they literally bleed into the uterine muscle causing extreme pain. This condition was first described by Rokitansky in 1860 and von Recklinghausen in 1896 (Benagiano, Brosens, Carrara, & Filippi, 2010).

Adenomyosis can be "focal" (localized to one area) or "diffuse" (spread throughout the uterine muscle). The "focal" form of adenomyosis is referred to an adenomyoma, and it is fairly easy to detect because it can usually be visualized on imaging studies. "Diffuse" adenomyosis is much more difficult to diagnose.

Adenomyosis can involve the entire thickness of the myometrium. Usually, the posterior wall of the uterus is the most severely affected. It differs from fibroids in that adenomyosis does not have clear, distinct borders. This makes removal of adenomyotic tissue very difficult.

Here are some interesting statistics about this uterine disorder:

- 80% of women with this disorder also have other uterine lesions with fibroids being the most common. In addition, it is difficult to differentiate between fibroids and adenomyosis.
- Polyps and adenocarcinoma occur more frequently in women with adenomyosis.
- 6-24% of women with adenomyosis also have endometriosis.
- 60% of women with endometrial carcinoma also have adenomyosis.
- Current diagnosis of this disorder prior to surgery is low, ranging from 3% to 26% (Taran, Stewart, & Brucker, 2013).

Adenomyosis has been reported to primarily affect middle-aged women and women who have had children. However, this line of thinking is beginning to change as more and more women are reporting symptoms of adenomyosis at a younger age and in those without children. The cause of this disorder is currently unknown as is the prevalence. Due to the lack of knowledge on this disorder, prevalence has been reported from 5% to 70% (Taran et al., 2013). At hysterectomy, the reported cases are around 20-30% (Taran et al., 2013). Additionally, according to Bromley, Shipp, and Benacerraf (2000), "the symptoms are so non-specific that the diagnosis is made preoperatively in fewer than half of patients undergoing hysterectomy" (Discussion section, para. 2).

So what's the difference between adenomyosis and endometriosis?

Adenomyosis and endometriosis are sometimes discussed together. There is good reason for this. At one time, adenomyosis was referred to as "endometriosis interna". That has now changed, but it does indicate some similarity between the two disorders. Also, in many cases, both disorders occur together.

While adenomyosis refers to endometrial tissue that has invaded the uterine muscle, endometriosis refers to endometrial tissue that has found its way outside of the uterine environment. It implants elsewhere in the pelvic cavity. Common sites of endometriosis include the bladder, the bowel, and the ovaries. To complicate diagnosis even further, the symptoms of endometriosis are quite similar to adenomyosis.

An interesting fact about endometriosis is pain level does not correlate with the amount of endometriosis present. Some women with very little endometriosis may suffer from debilitating pain while other women with severe endometriosis may have very little pain. It is important to know the amount of pain present does not indicate the severity of the disease.

According to the Endometriosis Foundation of America (EFA, 2015), endometriosis has been associated with auto-immune disease. However, there really is no consensus on what causes this disorder. It has been noted that a woman is seven times more likely to have endometriosis if her mother suffered from it (EFA, 2015).

The following are some interesting facts on endometriosis (EFA, 2015):

1. On average, it takes a woman ten years to obtain a correct diagnosis of endometriosis.

2. Approximately 176 million women suffer from this disorder worldwide.
3. Bowel symptoms of endometriosis are commonly misdiagnosed as irritable bowel syndrome (IBS).
4. Endometriosis is commonly misdiagnosed as pelvic inflammatory disease (PID).
5. Costs of the disorder are estimated to be about $22 billion annually.
6. Endometriosis is one of the top three causes of female infertility.

According to the EFA (2015), endometriosis can be easily misdiagnosed as adenomyosis, appendicitis, bowel obstruction, colon cancer, diverticulitis, ectopic pregnancy, fibroids, inflammatory bowel disease, irritable bowel syndrome, ovarian cancer, ovarian cysts, and pelvic inflammatory disease. Because this disorder can be so easily misdiagnosed, it is imperative the patient who experiences any of the above symptoms be seen by an expert in the field of endometriosis and adenomyosis.

More detailed information on the history of adenomyosis and endometriosis and how the two became separate disorders is addressed in the next chapter.

Chapter 2 - History of Adenomyosis and Endometriosis

Scientists have been aware of the presence of misplaced endometrial tissue for over 150 years. For decades, this tissue was referred to as an "adenomyoma", and its origin was not known. The first person to describe an "adenomyoma" in the literature was Carl von Rokitansky in 1860. Believing that the condition was cancerous, he called his finding "cystosarcoma adenoids uterinum".

In the late 1800's, Von Recklinghausen was able to distinguish two separate disease entities which today would refer to endometriosis and adenomyosis. He found some adenomyomas were inside the uterine muscle while others were outside the uterus. He noted the adenomyomas inside the uterine muscle appeared to have glands from the uterine mucosa while those outside the uterus did not.

In the early 1900's, Thomas Stephen Cullen, an American gynecologist, published findings on what we would call adenomyosis today. His diagnostic criteria included "lengthened menstrual periods...may be replaced by a continuous hemorrhagic discharge...great deal of pain" (Benagiano et al., 2010, Diagnosis section, para. 3). He divided the disorder into three different categories since he believed endometrial tissue was present not only in growths in the uterine wall, but also in growths that occurred outside the uterus (known as endometriosis today):

> Adenomyomas where the uterus maintains a normal shape
> Subperitoneal adenomyomas
> Submucosal adenomyomas

During his research on uteri that were affected by adenomyosis, Cullen noted a "uniformly enlarged uterus about four times the natural size. On opening it, I found that the increase in size was due to a diffuse thickening of the anterior wall" (Benangiano et al., 2010, Historical Perspectives section, para. 7).

During these early years, adenomyosis and endometriosis were included under the same diagnostic umbrella. Another physician, Lockyer, resisted the idea that adenomyomas located outside of the uterus contained endometrial tissue. He did, however, agree the abnormal growths occurred in many places, including the digestive tract, gallbladder, and kidneys. The subject of the source of the tissue was a point of contention for many years, but eventually Cullen's theory proved true.

In 1925, Frankl decided to name the invasion of endometrial tissue into the uterine muscle "adenomyosis uteri". He was also the first to clearly describe the difference between adenomyosis and adenomyomas. He also worked with Sampson to show the similarities seen between adenomyosis and endometriosis. While examining the uterine tissue of a fifty-year-old woman who had adenomyosis, he noted similarities between his findings and Sampson's findings. He stated "This observation reminds one of menstruating uterine mucosa on the surface of the ovary, first described by Sampson. By the courtesy of Sampson, I had an opportunity of studying the original slides, and I confirm that both in his and in my case, misplaced uterine glands were seen filled with blood, undoubtedly menstrual blood" (Benangiano et al., 2010, Definition section, para. 5). Two years later, Sampson named endometrial tissue found outside of the uterus as "endometriosis".

Recently, Kunz, Herbertz, Beil, Huppert, & Leyendecker (2007) used magnetic resonance imaging to determine that an area of the uterine wall called the junctional zone (JZ) may be of utmost importance in the diagnosis of endometriosis. The group determined that the thickness of the JZ directly correlated to the presence of endometriosis in the peritoneal cavity. These findings point to the fact that JZ abnormalities may be involved in both adenomyosis and endometriosis. Interestingly, a thickening of the JZ has also been linked to infertility.

Today, several radiological findings may suggest the presence of adenomyosis. According to Benagiano et al. (2010, Definition section, para. 6), a diagnosis of adenomyosis "should be restricted to the presence of glandular and stromal extensions of more than 2.5 mm below the endo-myometrial junction on low-power field." Since that time, new studies have shown a thickness of greater than 12 mm of the JZ can be considered diagnostic for adenomyosis (normal thickness is 5-12 mm).

Bird came up with the current definition of adenomyosis (as cited in Benagiano et al., 2010, Definition section, para.6):

> *"Adenomyosis may be defined as the benign invasion of endometrium into the myometrium, producing a diffusely enlarged uterus which microscopically exhibits ectopic non-neoplastic, endometrial glands and stroma surrounded by the hypertrophic and hyperplastic myometrium."*

As more studies are conducted, hopefully the current definition will be expanded to include more specifics on this disorder.

Chapter 3 - Anatomy and Function of the Uterus

In order to understand the problems associated with adenomyosis, it is important to understand the anatomy of the uterus. In this chapter, we will get into a more detailed description of the uterus and how hormones affect the proper functioning of the reproductive tract.

The uterus is located between the urinary bladder and the rectum. It is divided into three different parts: the fundus, the body of the uterus, and the cervix. The uterus is about 8 cm long, 5 cm wide, and 4 cm thick (Behera & Gest, 2011), and it is supported within the pelvis by broad ligaments. Within the body of the uterus, there are three distinct layers:

- The inner layer consists of glandular mucosa and is called the endometrium. This layer responds to the action of FSH and LH surges from the anterior pituitary gland. This layer also consists of two individual layers – the stratus functionalis and the stratus basalis. The stratum functionalis is involved in the thickening of this layer each month and is shed in the form of a menstrual period. This layer grows under the influence of estrogen and progesterone from the corpus luteum, a structure formed after the release of an egg each month. The stratum basalis is unresponsive to the cyclical hormonal levels.
- The thick and muscularis middle layer is called the myometrium and contains bundles of smooth muscle that contract rhythmically. This is the largest layer of the uterus and is the powerful muscular layer that contracts during childbirth and menstruation. It is regulated by oxytocin, prostaglandins, and the autonomic nervous system.
- The outer layer is called the perimetrium (also referred to the serosa layer). This layer envelops the uterus and consists of epithelial cells.

In addition to the above three layers, a distinct area can be seen between the endometrium and myometrium on magnetic resonance imaging (MRI). This is area is the previously discussed junctional zone, or JZ.

Blood is supplied to the uterus through the uterine artery. This artery branches off into to smaller arteries called radial arteries, and these supply blood to both the myometrium and endometrium. In the endometrium, they branch off even further to form basal and spiral arteries. The spiral arteries respond to female hormone levels, and when conception does not occur, these little arteries constrict resulting in a menstrual period.

The uterus can also have varying position within the pelvis. Sometimes the uterus tilts forward (anteflexion) or tilts backward (retroflexion). The anteflexed position is considered normal, and the retroflexed uterus is considered a normal variant and supposedly doesn't cause any issues for those who have it. Additionally, the uterus may also vary in size. During puberty and post-menopausal years, the uterus may be smaller than during childbearing years. It may also be smaller in women who have had no children in comparison to those who have given birth.

Day one of a woman's cycle is the first day of bleeding. Increases in follicle-stimulating hormone (FSH) and luteinizing hormone (LH) cause multiple ovarian follicles to start producing estrogen which, in turn, causes the endometrial lining to grow and thicken. Estrogen not only causes the endometrium to grow, but it also softens the cervix, produces vaginal secretions that allow the sperm to swim, and improves mood. At around day 14-15, a surge of LH causes the dominant follicle to rupture and release an egg. This egg makes its way down the fallopian tube. In the meantime, the remnants of the ruptured ovarian follicle (corpus luteum) begin to produce progesterone which prepares the uterine lining for fertilization. This hormone stops the buildup of the endometrium by counteracting the effects of estrogen. This part of the cycle is called the luteal phase, and it usually lasts anywhere from 12-14 days. If the egg is fertilized, human chorionic gonadotropin, or hCG, is secreted by the pituitary gland which increases the production of progesterone. If the egg is not fertilized, the progesterone level begins to fall which leads to the next menstrual cycle.

It is also important to know that there are three different kinds of estrogen. Estradiol, or E2, is the most potent estrogen followed by estrone (E1) and estriol (E3). E2 is the predominant form of estrogen during the reproductive years. E1 is the least abundant form of estrogen. It is predominately present during post-menopausal years and can be converted to E2 if needed. E3 is the type of estrogen produced by the placenta and is active during pregnancy.

The following are a list of the effects of estrogen and progesterone on a woman's body:

Estrogen

- Causes the endometrium to grown and thicken
- Stimulates the breast, possibly leading to fibrocystic disease or breast cancer
- Increases blood clotting
- Increases body fat
- Softens the cervix to allow sperm to enter the uterus and fertilize the egg
- Increases risk of endometrial cancer

Progesterone

- Prevents further growth of the endometrium, maintains pregnancy
- Helps protect against fibrocystic disease or breast cancer
- Normalizes blood clotting
- Helps to use fat as an energy source
- Maintains water balance by acting as a diuretic
- Prevents menstrual migraines
- Improves memory
- Increases sex drive

Both estrogen and progesterone need to be present in the right ratio to ensure the proper functioning of the reproductive tract. It has been noted in women with adenomyosis, the ratio of estrogen to progesterone is abnormal. There is not enough progesterone to counter the effects of estrogen. This condition is called estrogen dominance. As you can see from the information above, if insufficient progesterone is produced during the luteal phase of the cycle, this could potentially cause the endometrial lining to overgrow. This overgrowth of endometrial tissue could lead to endometriosis or adenomyosis. This is why the subject of estrogen dominance has been addressed by so many scientists and physicians regarding its role in the development of reproductive disorders. The subject of estrogen dominance will be discussed at length in Chapter 7.

In addition to the above effects, progesterone has a large impact on the functioning of the brain and the thymus gland. The thymus gland plays a very important role in the functioning of the immune system. This may explain why endometriosis is thought to develop due to an autoimmune process. In addition, progesterone is known to have impacts on the respiratory system and helps to support healthy growth of bones (Peat, 2014).

In addition to adenomyosis, there are other abnormalities that can occur in the uterus. The following is a list of some of these abnormalities along with a quick description of the problem. Some of these disorders have been seen in conjunction with adenomyosis.

Arcuate uterus – In this condition, the uterus had a slight indentation at the top. This is considered a normal uterine variant with no known adverse effects.

Asheman syndrome – In this syndrome, scarring inside the uterus occurs due to infection or surgery. Adhesions may be present.

Bicornuate uterus – This disorder is seen in about 1 out of every 200 women. Also called a "heart-shaped" uterus, this results from the failure of the upper part of the Müllerian ducts to fuse which leaves the upper portion of the uterus divided in two sections. This disorder does not appear to have any adverse effects on pregnancy.

Endometrial hyperplasia – Seen in women with adenomyosis, this is a condition where there is overgrowth of the endometrium.

Endometrial cancer – This form of cancer arises from the endometrial lining of the uterus.

Incompetent cervix – In this disorder, the cervix dilates too soon during pregnancy which results in pre-term labor or second trimester pregnancy loss.

Retroverted uterus – Seen in about twenty percent of women, the uterus is tipped backward toward the bowel rather than forward (normal). This altered position of the uterus is not associated with any reproductive problems.

Septate uterus – This is the most common congenital (present from birth) abnormality of the uterus. In this disorder, the uterus is divided partially or completely by a band of tissue or muscle, and this can result in repeat cases of miscarriage. Thankfully, this condition can be corrected through surgery. It is seen in about 1 out of 45 women.

Unicornuate uterus – In this disorder, only one half of the uterus forms. The uterus is only about ½ the size of a normal uterus, and only one fallopian tube and ovary are present. This rare disorder occurs in about 1 in every 1000 women.

Uterine cancer – Risk factors for this type of cancer include age over 50, obesity, taking unopposed estrogen (estrogen without progesterone), and family history of this type of cancer. Symptoms include an abnormal vaginal discharge, abnormal vaginal bleeding, pelvic pain, and/or pelvic pressure.

Uterine didelphys – This disorder occurs when the Müllerian ducts fail to fuse and results in two separate uteri. Many times, there is also a separate cervix and vagina associated with each uterus. Also referred to as a double uterus, this disorder occurs in about 1 out of every 350 women.

Uterine fibroid – These are benign masses that form from the myometrial layer of the uterus and may be present in women with adenomyosis.

Uterine polyp – These benign growths are found inside the uterus are due to overgrowth of the endometrium. They may be present in women with adenomyosis.

Chapter 4 - Symptoms of Adenomyosis

The following is a comprehensive list of all the possible symptoms of adenomyosis. Some women experience many of the symptoms below while other women don't have any symptoms at all. The pain associated with this disorder may increase over time may become debilitating.

In my case, I had about seventy-five percent of these symptoms. The most severe issue for me was the severe abdominal cramping. My periods were heavy and long, and I felt horrible, but I don't think that was the worst of it for me. I have heard many women talk about how they had to change their pad/tampon every hour due to the heavy bleeding. I have also heard stories about how some women had to wear two pads at a time, and the blood still seeped through on their clothing.

During my period, I suffered terribly with constipation. I had a retroflexed uterus, and even though this position of the uterus isn't supposed to cause any issues, I sometimes wonder if the retroflexion played a role in the constipation. A retroflexed uterus tilts backward toward the rectum, and if the uterus enlarges during an attack of adenomyosis, wouldn't that place extra pressure on the bowel? The cramping pain and constipation were so bad in my case I actually thought I had a bowel obstruction. I still wonder that to this day. I also wonder if women who had an anteflexed uterus suffer from more bladder issues since the uterus is tilted forward toward the bladder. These are just my own thoughts. I haven't found any discussion about this issue in the scientific literature, but I would love to see a study on this aspect of the disorder.

Please keep in mind that not everyone will have all of these symptoms, and not everyone will experience the symptoms to the same degree.

Heavy menstrual bleeding (menorrhagia), also called "flooding"
Severe abdominal cramping (dysmenorrhea), sometimes can be as severe as the last stage of labor
Enlarged, bulky, and heavy uterus (often doubling or tripling in size)
Tenderness during a pelvic exam
Severe bloating
Nausea and vomiting
A "bearing down" sensation
Heaviness and pain in the legs
Pain in the lower back
Bleeding between periods
Continuous bloody discharge (spotting)
Painful intercourse
Pressure on the bladder
Frequent urination
Painful bowel movements during menstruation

Alternating constipation and diarrhea (can be confused with irritable bowel syndrome)
Passing large blood clots during menstruation
Prolonged menstrual bleeding (8 to 14 days, sometimes longer)
Chronic anemia
Heart palpitations due to anemia
Dizziness due to anemia
Depression and/or anxiety
Infertility
Miscarriage
Predisposed to myometrial ectopic pregnancy

As can be seen from the list above, adenomyosis can have a serious impact on the quality of a woman's life. For those who haven't had to deal with adenomyosis, all I can say is please don't judge someone unless you have walked in their shoes. I don't think anyone can understand the amount of pain, fatigue, blood loss, and depression that is involved in this disorder unless you have actually been through it.

Chapter 5 - What are the Risk Factors?

Although little is known about this disorder, there are a few factors that appear to put women at risk for adenomyosis. Some of these factors, such as age, may be changing as this disorder is reportedly being seen more and more in younger women.

Age – Years ago, adenomyosis was thought to occur primarily in older women in their 40's or 50's. A possibility for the increase in this disorder at older age could be due to a woman's repeated exposure to estrogens. However, this line of thinking is beginning to change. Discoveries with junctional zone abnormalities of the uterus through MRI have shown chronic pelvic pain and heavy menstrual bleeding in younger women may actually be due to adenomyosis. According to Taran et al., (2013) studies "suggest that the clinical age at presentation of adenomyosis may be significantly earlier than previously thought and that early-stage adenomyosis might present a different clinical phenotype compared to late-stage disease" (Risk Factors section, para. 1).

Multiple pregnancies – Women who have had multiple children appear to have a higher rate of adenomyosis as opposed to those who have had no children (Taran et al., 2013). Also, Parazzini et al. (1997) report the greater number of births, the higher the risk of adenomyosis. This could be due to the disruption between the endometrium and myometrium during pregnancy, or it could also be due to pregnancy hormonal levels.

Prior surgery on the uterus – Studies have repeatedly shown that prior uterine surgery may possibly play a role in the development of adenomyosis. The theory is that any kind of uterine trauma that could break the endometrial/myometrial barrier may lead to the infiltration of the endometrium into the myometrium. The procedures that may lead to this problem include cesarean section (C-section), fibroid and/or polyp removal, abortions, miscarriages, spontaneous abortions, and D&C. In fact, several studies show that D&Cs may be linked to higher rates of adenomyosis (Taran et al., 2013). In addition, another study showed a higher rate in women who had cesarean section (Taran et al, 2013). Interestingly, Panganamamula et al. (2004) report adenomyosis has been reported to occur after endometrial ablations. However, studies have been inconsistent. Other studies have not been able to confirm these findings.

Antidepressant use – Use of Prozac may increase prolactin levels and put a woman at increased risk for adenomyosis. See "Hyperprolactinemia" in Chapter 6 for more information.

Treatment with Tamoxifen – In women treated with Tamoxifen for breast cancer, an increased incidence of adenomyosis has been noted (Taran et al., 2013).

Although there appears to be some factors that put women at risk for adenomyosis, clearly more research is needed. Interestingly, studies so far have shown that smoking, birth control pills, and IUDs have no association with the development of adenomyosis. However, the studies are few and far between, so I take these results with a grain of salt. Since adenomyosis appears to be dependent on estrogen, I find it hard to believe that birth control pills in particular to have no effect on this disorder. I strongly encourage more researchers to develop well-controlled studies to give us more information on the cause of this uterine disorder.

Chapter 6 - So What Goes Wrong?

The theory that has been accepted for many years is adenomyosis is caused by some kind of trauma that breaks the barrier between the endometrium and myometrium. However, this theory has not been proven. Other studies have shown other factors may be at play.

Hyperprolactinemia

Hyperprolactinemia, or high levels of prolactin, may play a role as several animal studies have shown adenomyosis occurs in this state. Sengupta et al. (2013) expanded on this idea in a study by looking at the role of fluoxetine (Prozac) as a possible cause of adenomyosis since fluoxetine causes an increase in prolactin secretion. They were able to show a significant increase in prolactin levels in mice when treated with fluoxetine, and histological examination of the uteri showed evidence of adenomyosis. It is unknown if hyperprolactinemia is a factor in adenomyosis development in the human body, and further studies are needed to confirm the findings in this animal study.

Autoimmune factors

Endometriosis is thought to have autoimmune factors that play into the disorder. Because of this, Ota, Igarashi, Hatazawa, and Tanaka (1998) looked at autoimmune factors in adenomyosis. They found significant abnormal immune responses, and they specifically noted autoantibodies in the peripheral blood of women with adenomyosis.

Hyperperistalsis

Kunz et al. (2007) suggest hyperperistalsis (abnormal contractions) of the uterine muscle may play a role in both adenomyosis and endometriosis. The researchers noted in women with endometriosis, hyperperistalsis occurred during the early and mid-follicular phases and mid luteal phase of the menstrual cycle. In the late follicular state, the contractions became arrhythmic and convulsive in women with endometriosis.

Beta Catenin

In a study done at Michigan State University (Oh et al., 2013), the protein beta-catenin was found to play a possible role in the development of adenomyosis. Beta-catenin was first discovered in the early 1990's, and this substance was found to play an integral role in the formation of complex animal tissues. Specifically, it is involved in cell adhesion formations in the maintenance and growth of the epithelium. It helps to regulate the growth and apoptosis of epithelial cells (Beta-catenin, 2015). Apoptosis refers to programmed cell death. If a cell is damaged or not useful, the body automatically tells it to "self-destruct". This is a necessary function of the human body. If the apoptosis "signal" is turned off, cells would reproduce unchecked which can lead to a whole host of problems. Cancer is a perfect example of faulty apoptosis. Interestingly, mutations (or shutting off the "signal" for apoptosis) of beta-catenin have been noted in many different cancers such as basal cell carcinoma, prostate cancer, and medulloblastoma (Beta-catenin, 2015). More research in this area needs to be done to determine the exact mechanism of action of beta-catenin in the development of adenomyosis.

Vascular Endothelial Growth Factor (VEGF)

VEGF has been found to have an increased expression in women with adenomyosis. This substance is a potent factor in angiogenesis. Angiogenesis refers to the formation of new blood vessels from pre-existing ones. This process is necessary when a wound is healing, but it can be problematic in other diseases such as cancer.

The production of VEGF is known to be enhanced by estradiol. In addition, it is known to be expressed in endometriosis cells. According to Rocha, Reis, & Taylor (2013), "Endometriomas and red implants show the highest concentrations of VEGF" (Results section, para. 3). Another interesting finding is pro-angiogenic factors, including VEGF, are seen in increased levels in the peritoneal (abdominal) fluid of women who suffer from endometriosis. (Rocha et al., 2013).

Some anti-angiogenic drugs are currently being tested for possible use in adenomyosis patients in the future. Bevacizumab inhibits VEGF, and this drug showed some promising results in mice studies (Rocha et al., 2013). Other possible anti-angiogenic drugs include Sorafenib and Romidepsin. Retinoic acid has been shown to have anti-angiogenic effects and has been shown to be useful in mouse studies. Progestogens have been shown to suppress the transcription of VEGF, and this may be one reason progestogens have been useful in the treatment of both endometriosis and adenomyosis. The statin drugs have also been shown to have anti-angiogenic properties. Atorvastatin has been shown to inhibit COX2 and VEGF in endometriosis cells, and Lovastatin has been shown to inhibit angiogenesis (Rocha et al., 2013).

COX2 and MMP2

In a study by Tokyol, Aktepe, Dilek, Sahin, and Arioz (2009), the expression of cyclo-oxygenase (COX2) and matrix metalloproteinase (MMP2) were investigated in women with adenomyosis. The group found the expression of both were higher during the follicular and secretory phases of the menstrual cycle than in women without adenomyosis.

COX2 is an enzyme that is directly involved in inflammation. It is responsible for the production of prostaglandins which cause both inflammation and pain. This may be part of the reason NSAIDS are a possible treatment as NSAIDS block the production of prostaglandins.

MMP2 is involved in the breakdown of the extracellular matrix. It also plays an important role in angiogenesis and promotes the mobilization of vascular endothelial growth factor (VEGF). This substance is known to be involved in the breakdown of the endometrium during menstruation. It is also interesting that increased levels of MMP2 are seen in melanoma, breast, and ovarian cancers, and that these increased levels indicate a poor prognosis for the patient.

HOX gene

A study performed by Taylor et al. (2000) looked at the expression of the HOX gene in the regulation of the development of the endometrium. They found that the gene expression was abnormal. This could indicate a problem with endometrial development at the molecular level.

Hypoestrogenism (estrogen dominance)

The most interesting finding is reported by Campo, Campo and Benagiano (2012), and having suffered through years of adenomyosis, I find this particular report most interesting. In adenomyosis, interleukin-6 (IL-6) is overexpressed. They report this could lead to increased estrogen receptor expression. They continue to say that estrogen and progesterone expression in women with adenomyosis are different than in women with normal uteri. In addition, they note because there is overexpression of cytochrome P450 in women with adenomyosis, this can contribute to overexpression of local estrogen production. Also, a defect in progesterone receptor sites was observed. This could explain why estrogen dominance is noted in women with adenomyosis.

Another interesting study regarding estrogen expression in adenomyosis tissue was performed in 2014 by Yamanaka et al. The group notes aromatase and estrogen sulphatase levels are higher in adenomyotic tissue. Aromatase is an enzyme that is involved in the conversion of androgens to estrogen. Scientists are looking into ways to block aromatase as a way of inhibiting the production of estrogen. Yamanaka et al. (2014) states this high level of aromatase suggests a higher sensitivity to estrogen in adenomyotic tissue. Also, they note adenomyotic cells appear to be resistant to apoptosis. The group goes on to say some progestins appear to improve symptoms, so they decided to look at the effects of two progesterone agents on adenomyotic tissue. One exciting finding was both endogenous progesterone (progesterone produced in the body) and dienogest (synthetic progesterone) increased apoptosis of adenomyotic cells. They conclude both endogenous progesterone and dienogest "directly inhibit cellular proliferation and also induce apoptosis in human adenomyotic stromal cells" (Comment section, para. 4). The researchers suggest dienogest may be useful in the treatment of adenomyosis.

Occurrence of Other Uterine Disorders with Adenomyosis

Kunz et al. (2007) state adenomyosis and endometriosis may be different forms of the same disease since both involve displaced endometrial tissue. In addition, this same group determined that in a group of women with known endometriosis, 70% also had adenomyosis as compared to a normal control group in which only 9% of women were found to have the disorder. Although this same group of researchers found a significantly higher rate of adenomyosis in women with endometriosis, Bazot et al. (2001) only found 27 percent of women with endometriosis also had adenomyosis. The discrepancy can be blamed on the different imaging criteria that are currently being used to diagnose the disorders.

An interesting study done by Millischer et al. (2013) showed the presence of adenomyosis could be a marker of deep intestinal endometriosis. They found 76% of patients with diffuse adenomyosis had more than one deep intestinal lesion as compared to the control group without adenomyosis. Also, if the adenomyosis was focal and located in the posterior section of the uterus, the number of intestinal lesions was greater. Eighty-seven percent with this type of adenomyosis had three or more intestinal lesions.

Adenomyosis is also commonly seen with uterine fibroids. A study by Shrestha and Sedai (2012) looked at the differences between women with adenomyosis alone and those with uterine fibroids. They found women with adenomyosis only had higher levels of chronic pelvic pain and a smaller uterus. The women who had fibroids only had less pelvic pain and a larger uterus. They suggested that if a woman presents with fibroids, a small uterus, and chronic pelvic pain, the physician should suspect the co-existence of adenomyosis with fibroids.

As you can see, there are many different factors at play in the development of adenomyosis. Although these studies give us a little more insight, much more research needs to be done. Well-controlled trials are needed to verify or disprove the findings discussed in this chapter.

Chapter 7 - So What is Estrogen Dominance?

Estrogen and progesterone need to be in a delicate balance in a woman's body for proper functioning of the reproductive tract. Estrogen dominance is a condition in which the progesterone to estrogen ratio is too low. In other words, there is not enough progesterone present to counter the effects of estrogen. This can lead to a whole host of problems with the most notable being breast cancer. Sadly, this condition is not generally recognized by mainstream physicians. Rather, it is a condition that is usually observed and treated by natural health practitioners. I include it here because I do believe that a hormonal imbalance plays a role in adenomyosis, and recent studies have found that adenomyosis is indeed estrogen-dependent.

The abnormal ratio between progesterone and estrogen is typically not picked up by routine laboratory testing as the ratio between these two hormones is not usually calculated. In estrogen dominance, both estrogen and progesterone levels can be in the "normal" range, but the ratio of progesterone to estrogen can be out of range. The following is a measurement of my levels several years ago when I was struggling with some gynecological issues. The test was performed at ZRT Laboratories.

> Estradiol   2.3   In range (normal is 1.3-3.3)
> Progesterone 154   In range (normal is 75-270
> Ratio: Pg/E2 67   **Out of range (normal is 100-500)**

Note: Pg stands for progesterone, E2 stands for estradiol

As you can see, this condition can be easily missed if the ratio of progesterone to estrogen is not calculated. Hormonal balance has largely been underestimated in the past as a cause of gynecological disorders. Today, the prevalence of this condition in the U.S. has been reported to be close to 50 percent.

It has been reported that from age 35 to age 50, the level of estrogen in a woman's body will decline by about 35% while during that same period of time, the progesterone level will decline by 75% (Biomedic Labs Rx, What is Estrogen Dominance section, para. 3). So, as you can see, estrogen dominance is of utmost concern as a woman ages.

The causes of estrogen dominance include menopause, polycystic ovarian syndrome, anovulation, luteal insufficiency, exposure to xenoestrogens, exposure to synthetic progestins (birth control pills), poor diet (including a lack of omega-3 fatty acids, excess refined carbohydrates, and low fiber), lack of exercise, certain medications, stress, an impaired immune system, obesity, ovarian tumors, adrenal fatigue, and thyroid disorders.

Anovulation occurs when a woman does not ovulate. If an egg is not released during a cycle, the corpus luteum is not present; therefore, no progesterone will be produced. Luteal insufficiency is a condition where the corpus luteum doesn't produce enough progesterone. The result of both of these conditions is an estrogen dominant condition in the woman.

The following is a list of possible symptoms that have been associated with estrogen dominance. This is not a comprehensive list.

Adenomyosis
Allergies
Anxiety
Asthma
Auto-immune disorders
Bloating
Blood clots
Breast cancer
Cold hands and feet
Cravings for carbohydrates
Decreased sex drive
Depression
Digestive problems
Dry eyes
Endometrial cancer
Endometrial polyps
Endometriosis
Fatigue
Fibrocystic breasts
Foggy thinking
Hair loss
Headaches (including migraines, often premenstrual)
Heavy menstrual periods (menorrhagia)
Hypoglycemia (low blood sugar)
Infertility
Irregular periods
Irritability
Insomnia
Memory loss
Mineral deficiencies (magnesium and zinc)
Mood swings
Osteoporosis
Ovarian cysts
Painful menstrual periods (dysmenorrhea)
Pre-menopausal bone loss
Premenstrual syndrome (PMS)
Prolonged menstruation
Polycystic ovarian syndrome (PCOS)
Sinus congestion

Slow metabolism
Spotting between periods (breakthrough bleeding)
Unwanted hair growth
Uterine cancer
Uterine fibroids
Weight gain in the abdomen, hips, and thighs

What Can We Do to Balance Hormone Levels?

The following list includes many different ways to ensure we have a proper progesterone to estrogen ratio:

1. Take a high quality multivitamin and mineral supplement to ensure you are getting the proper basic nutrients.
2. Educate yourself on how to eat a well-balanced diet that will also promote hormonal balance. See Chapter 12 for more information on this subject.
3. Be sure to get plenty of fiber since estrogen is excreted through the bowel.
4. Include a high quality omega-3 supplement to your vitamin regime. See Chapter 15 for an in-depth discussion of omega-3 fatty acids.
5. Use a high quality bioidentical progesterone cream. Dr. John Lee offers a great product, and it can be found and purchased at www.johnleemd.com.
6. If overweight, make it a goal to lose the excess body fat. Exercise at least three times per week, and be sure to include strength training.
7. Reduce your stress level. Get rid of things in your life that aren't absolutely necessary, and learn to say "no".
8. Consider doing a detoxification cleanse. The liver processes estrogen and eliminates toxins, and if the liver is sluggish, this may increase the problem of estrogen dominance. A detoxification cleanse is well worth the effort. See Chapter 13 for more information.
9. Quit smoking.
10. Lower exposure to xenoestrogens. See Chapter 14 for more information.
11. Be careful with hormone replacement therapy (HRT). Taking unopposed estrogen (estrogen without progesterone) can lead to estrogen dominance and can increase your risk of cancer. Do your research before moving to HRT.
12. Cut down on coffee consumption. Studies have shown women who consume four to five cups of coffee per day have 70% more circulating estrogen in their bodies as compared to those women who consume less than one cup per day (Lam, 2015b).

Chapter 8 - How Is Adenomyosis Diagnosed?

Again, not enough research has been done on this uterine disorder when it comes to diagnosis. Benagiano et al. (2009) state "…today a clinical diagnosis of adenomyosis is considered practically impossible" (Clinical Diagnosis section, para. 1). There is no consensus on what the criteria should be used to diagnose a woman with adenomyosis. In hysterectomy specimens, most physicians agree that if there is endometrial intrusion of >2.5 mm into the myometrium, a diagnosis of adenomyosis should be made. Nevertheless, some irregularities such as JZ thickness have been observed on ultrasound and MRI and may indicate adenomyosis. The next chapter discusses recent findings regarding the JZ.

Hysterosalpingography – On the night before the procedure, the patient may be given a laxative, and on the day of the procedure, a sedative may be given. The patient is placed on her back with her feet in stirrups. A speculum is placed in the vagina, and a catheter in threaded through the cervix. The speculum is then removed, and a contrast medium is introduced into the uterus through the catheter. This medium enables the physician to more clearly visualize the wall of the uterus. X-rays are taken. When the physician is finished, the catheter is removed, and the patient is generally allowed to go home right after the procedure. The entire procedure lasts about thirty minutes.

Although this test may be done to rule out other abnormalities, it is not generally suggested for use in a diagnosis of adenomyosis due to its low sensitivity and specificity. However, Molinas and Campo (2006) suggest it could be useful since the endometrium may appear irregular with cystic lesions and abnormal vascularization. It appears this procedure would only be of use if the technician/doctor were heavily educated and experienced in the diagnosis of adenomyosis.

I underwent a hysterosalpinography during the years that I struggled with adenomyosis; however, the reason for the exam was due to the presence of a uterine polyp. I did not have any discomfort during the actual test even though I was told I might have some minor cramping when they injected the contrast medium into the uterus. I did, however, experience severe cramping about thirty minutes after the test while I was on my way home and in the middle of rush hour traffic. I did not expect this at all and was not warned that this might happen. Thankfully, my husband was driving at the time. I felt like I had to defecate, so my husband stopped at a fast food restaurant. I had a large bowel movement, and the pain decreased almost immediately (please note that I was not given a laxative the night before the test). I suspect the contrast medium irritated the uterus, and I had a delayed reaction. I don't want to scare anyone from having this test, but I feel it's very important for women to be prepared. If you have adenomyosis and have this test, you may want to wait in the office for about 30 minutes or so to make sure you don't have a delayed reaction. It may also be advisable to have some kind of pain relief available just in case, and you may want to ask for a laxative the night before the test if one is not offered to you.

Hysteroscopy – This procedure is used to look at the lining of the uterus and can be done using either local or general anesthesia. First, the patient is placed in stirrups. A small, thin scope is inserted into the vagina and then moved through the cervix and into the uterus. Gas or liquid is introduced into the uterus through the hysteroscope so the physician can better visualize the uterine lining. During the procedure, the doctor can take a biopsy, remove fibroids, or remove uterine polyps if necessary. A hysteroscopy takes about thirty minutes, and it is usually done on an outpatient basis. Within the first twenty-four hours of recovery, the patient may experience some mild cramping and/or light bleeding. Sadly, this procedure is generally not useful in the diagnosis of adenomyosis since it does not look at the thickness of the uterine wall, but it may be a good place to start as it can rule out other causes of abnormal menstrual bleeding. Interestingly, Wortman and Daggett (2001) report that hysteroscopy may be useful in women who have undergone a failed endometrial ablation and resection.

My experience with this procedure is about the same as a D&C. I was given a general anesthetic, and the procedure was done in a hospital. I had mild cramping and light bleeding as expected, but I was back to work after missing two days – one for surgery and one for recovery. In general, I found it very easy to recover from a hysteroscopy.

2D/3D transvaginal ultrasound (TVS) – This test is done with a full bladder. The patient lies on her back with her feet in stirrups. The transvaginal probe is covered with a condom and some lubricating gel. The probe is placed inside the vagina, and the technician moves it around a bit to take pictures of the reproductive organs.

Adenomyosis can be detected by TVS if the technician/doctor is knowledgeable regarding adenomyosis as this procedure is highly observer-dependent. In a review of adenomyosis by Benagiano et al. (2010, Transvaginal Sonography section, para. 4), they state "TVS should be favored as the primary diagnostic tool, although substantial experience and specific training is required to make sonography a useful diagnostic tool" (Transvaginal sonography section, para. 4). According to Streuli et al. (2014, Section 1.1, para.1)), red flags include "globular uterus, asymmetry of uterine walls, poorly defined junctional zone, poorly defined focus of abnormal myometrial echotexture, distorted and heterogeneous myometrial echotexture, myometrial linear striations and myometrial cysts". In another article by Bromley et al. (2000, Discussion section, para. 11)., the signs to look for on ultrasound include a "mottled heterogeneous appearing myometrium, a globular asymmetric uterus, small myometrial lucent areas, and an indistinct endometrial stripe." Although encouraging, these different studies use different criteria to diagnose adenomyosis; therefore, the data so far has not been too helpful. It needs to be noted though that Exacoustos et al. (2011) report the presence of myometrial cysts on a 2D TVS can indicate adenomyosis with an accuracy of 78 percent and a specificity of 98%. In addition, the same group states adenomyosis can be detected on a 3D TVS with an accuracy of 85 percent if the JZ difference in thickness is >4mm. This test is not recommended in cases of an enlarged uterus or fibroids.

I have had many trans-vaginal ultrasounds during my battle with adenomyosis. Sadly, even though I had this test numerous times, adenomyosis was never picked up using this test. However, I struggled with this disorder twenty to thirty years ago, so they really didn't have the knowledge that they have today. TVS is fairly easy and painless overall. The worst part for me was having a full bladder. This is especially a problem if the office is running behind on appointments and you have to wait. To deal with this problem, make sure the receptionist knows that you have a full bladder and that you can't wait too long. They should understand and work with you. Also, on a couple of occasions, the technician tried to get a good image of my ovaries, and she pushed the probe far to the side which caused some pain. If it is uncomfortable, be sure to tell the technician. Don't be quiet – you are your own advocate in these situations.

Magnetic Resonance Imaging – This imaging technique has become extremely valuable for adenomyosis diagnosis. On T-2 weighted magnetic resonance images, the JZ can be visualized quite well. On MRI, there are three distinct zones that can be identified in the uterine wall. The endometrium has a high signal intensity. Underneath this layer is an area of low signal intensity which is JZ. The myometrium has a medium signal intensity. A normal junctional zone is about 5-8 mm wide, and widening of this area to 12 mm or more suggests adenomyosis is present. MRI has been found to be the most useful test for detecting adenomyosis when fibroids or other abnormalities are present.

According to Novellas et al. (2011), the presence of microcysts within the junctional zone or myometrium are signs of the presence of adenomyosis. These cysts can vary from 2 to 7 mm in diameter. However, according to this same group, these cysts can only be detected in about fifty percent of cases. An adenomyoma is easier to detect, but it must be differentiated from a uterine fibroid. Dueholm et al. report the use of both TVS and MRI give the most accurate results in the diagnosis of adenomyosis.

Since I suffered from adenomyosis from 1990-2007, information about thickening of the junctional zone was not available to the physicians at that time; therefore, an MRI was never ordered in my case. Hopefully that is all changing now. This new knowledge about the junctional zone should prompt more physicians to move to MRI if they suspect adenomyosis.

Chapter 9 - Junctional Zone Abnormalities

Recently, the junctional zone has been of great interest with regard to adenomyosis. As described earlier, this area is the small layer between the endometrium and the myometrium. The JZ has been observed to contract in the non-pregnant uterus, and it is believed to be involved in the transport of sperm into the uterus to fertilize the egg (Novellas et al., 2011). In general, there have been consistent observations that a thicker than normal junctional zone points to adenomyosis. This thickening is usually seen in the posterior wall of the uterus and is an encouraging finding as this may help to diagnose the condition prior to hysterectomy.

The thickness of the JZ usually ranges from 5 to 8 mm in normal, healthy women. As previously stated, a JZ thickness of 12 mm or more could be an indication of adenomyosis. Reinhold et al. (1996) showed a thickness of more than 12 mm is a strong indicator of the presence of infiltration of the endometrium into the myometrium. Additionally, Novellas et al. (2011) state a thickness of greater than 12 mm indicates adenomyosis with an accuracy of 85 percent and a specificity of 96 percent. This thickening can possibly be seen on ultrasound IF the technologist and the doctor are well trained to detect this abnormality. According to Benangiano et al. (2010), MRI should be used to confirm the diagnosis. If the entire JZ is involved, the diagnosis is diffuse adenomyosis whereas if only a portion of the JZ is involved, the diagnosis is focal adenomyosis (Novellas et al., 2011).

The thickening of the JZ reaches its maximum width during menstruation due to the effects of hormones (Novellas et al., 2011). Benagiano et al (2010, Adenomyosis section, para. 2) points out that "It is advisable to perform MRI for the diagnosis of adenomyosis after menstruation, as menstrual contraction waves can mimic abnormal JZ thickening."

However, there is a complicating factor here. As women age, the JZ normally becomes thicker. In fact, the junctional zone cannot be delineated in about thirty percent of post-menopausal women (Novellas et al., 2011). It should also be noted that the JZ is poorly identified via MRI during premenarche and during pregnancy. Benangiano et al. (2010) discuss in a review of adenomyosis that the term "junctional zone hyperplasia" refers to JZ thickening without any other signs of adenomyosis. They point out this problem of JZ thickening as women age and concluded the term "junctional zone hyperplasia" should only apply to women less than 35 years of age. Gordts, Brosens, Fusi, Benagiano, & Brosens (2008) clarifies this problem even further and even developed a classification system, although it still needs to be validated. The classification system is outlined below:

- Simple JZ hyperplasia – a junctional zone thickness between 8 mm and 12 mm in women 35 years old or less.

- Partial or diffuse adenomyosis – a junctional zone thickness > or =12 mm, high signal intensity myometrial cysts, and involvement of the outer myometrium
- Adenomyoma – myometrial mass, low signal intensity, indistinct border

A couple of other studies have looked further into the thickness of the JZ and the estrogen receptors of the JZ in adenomyosis. These studies are interesting and possibly very useful. I will mention them here as they may give researchers ideas for future studies.

A study by Dueholm et al. (2001) looked at the differences in the thickness in the JZ of the entire uterus since the thickness can be different at different locations. They termed this the "junctional zone differential" and found if the difference in thickness throughout the entire JZ was more than 5 mm, it indicated adenomyosis more effectively than an overall thickness of 12 mm or greater.

Reinhold et al. (1996) looked at the thickness of the JZ in relation to the thickness of the myometrium. They found a ratio of >40% was also indicative of adenomyosis.

Another interesting study looked at the estrogen receptor sites at the endometrial-myometrial interface (EMI, also known as the JZ). Wang, Zhang and Duan (2010) determined the expression of estrogen receptor-α at the endometrial-myometrial interface in adenomyosis patients as compared to normal patients varied significantly at certain stages. They concluded that "The loss of periodic expression of ERα in myometrium of EMI of adenomyosis may be associated with an abnormal regulation of estrogen in adenomyosis" (Abstract).

These findings are very encouraging as they give much more information about the disorder, but the findings need to be confirmed. I encourage researchers to continue these studies as they will offer much more insight into adenomyosis which may lead to ways to treat it more effectively.

Chapter 10 - How is Adenomyosis Treated?

Although there is currently no cure for adenomyosis, there are many ways to manage the disorder. In this chapter, we will address the surgical and pharmacological avenues that can be taken in an attempt to reduce symptoms of adenomyosis.

Surgical treatments

Adenomyomectomy – This procedure involves cutting into the uterine wall and removing the adenomyotic lesions. It is also referred to as a wedge resection of the uterine wall. This surgery has been linked to spontaneous uterine rupture during pregnancy, so a group led by Osada improved it by using a double-flap or triple-flap method when closing the uterine wall after the procedure (see Osada procedure). Excision of adenomyosis will only be useful if the area of adenomyosis is focal and contained, but even in this circumstance, the effectiveness is only reported at 50% (Taran et al., 2013). Fedele et al. (1993) report a high rate of spontaneous abortion after this procedure. In addition, there is a high rate of recurrence of adenomyosis with this procedure. However, another study showed the use of this surgery plus treatment with GnRH analogs produced statistically significant symptom relief.

Dilation and curettage (D&C) – This surgery is usually one of the first steps in treating heavy and/or abnormal menstrual bleeding. It is performed under general anesthesia usually on an outpatient basis. The surgeon first dilates the cervix and then used a small spoon shaped instrument to scrape or suction out the entire contents of the uterus. By doing this, he/she may also remove any polyps or fibroids that are found. If there is concern for cancer or endometrial hyperplasia, a piece of the endometrial tissue will be sent to a pathology lab for examination. After the procedure, there may be some cramping or spotting, but the patient is usually up and moving a few hours later.

I have undergone a D&C many times due to heavy bleeding. The first time resulted in fairly significant cramping; however, the nurse in the recovery room gave me plenty of pain medication. Also, I did have some bleeding, but this resolved within a day. Overall, in my opinion, this surgery is fairly easy to tolerate, and recovery is quick.

Endometrial ablation – This surgical procedure destroys the endometrial layer of the uterus. It is not recommended for women who still want to have children. No incision is needed as tools for the procedure are inserted into the uterus through the vagina and cervix. It is done under general anesthesia. There are several different ways to perform an ablation. The possible methods used in this procedure include microwave energy, high-energy radiofrequencies, electrosurgery, cryosurgery, or heated liquids. Once the cervix is dilated, the method of choice is used to "burn" the endometrial lining.

After the surgery is completed, patients can expect some mild cramping and a watery or bloody discharge for a few days. It is possible to become pregnant after this procedure, but the pregnancy is usually miscarried. Therefore, it is imperative the patient use some form of birth control after undergoing an ablation.

An endometrial ablation may be beneficial to women who have superficial adenomyosis; however, those with deep adenomyosis may fail an ablation. In fact, according to Loffer (1995), 8 to 10 percent of women with adenomyosis will fail an endometrial ablation. In addition, Pagedas, Bae, and Perkins (1995) reported that in hysterectomies of women who failed an ablation, 75 percent were found to have adenomyosis. Also, a large study on ablation failures was conducted at the Mayo Clinic. This study showed that women with adenomyosis had an increased failure risk and required either repeat ablation or hysterectomy (Taran et al., 2013). If the woman has deep adenomyosis and has failed an ablation, hysterectomy is usually indicated. According to Benangiano et al. (2010), deep adenomyosis is considered if the adenomyotic tissue has penetrated 2.5 cm or more into the myometrium.

I underwent an endometrial ablation, and it failed. The procedure itself was fairly easy and similar to a D&C. However, I began to bleed heavily within 24 hours of having the surgery. After my hysterectomy, I found out I had deep, diffuse adenomyosis, and this explained the reason for the failed ablation.

Hysterectomy – In the past, a hysterectomy was usually performed through an abdominal incision. Thankfully, due to surgical advancements, a hysterectomy is now done vaginally or through the use of a laparoscope which dramatically reduces recovery time. The average time to perform a hysterectomy is two hours, and there are several different types of hysterectomy as detailed below:

- **Total abdominal hysterectomy** – the uterus and cervix are removed.
- **Vaginal hysterectomy** – the uterine tissue is removed through the vagina.
- **Supracervical hysterectomy** – the uterus is removed, but the cervix remains.
- **Laparoscopic hysterectomy** – the uterus and cervix are removed through the vagina with the help of a laparoscope.
- **Laparoscopic supracervical hysterectomy** – the uterine tissue is removed through the laparoscopic incisions.

- **Radical hysterectomy** – this type is more extensive than the total because it also removes the upper part of the vagina. It is usually done if cancer is present.
- **Oophorectomy** - removal of the ovaries. It is usually done if there is a history of cancer or if cancer is present.
- **Salpingo-oophorectomy** – removal of the ovaries and fallopian tubes. It is usually done if there is a history of cancer or if cancer is present.

This surgery has been the only way to diagnose and treat adenomyosis for more than a century. According to a study by Furuhashi, Miyabe, Katsumata, Oda, and Imai (1998), women who have adenomyosis have a higher risk of bladder injury during a hysterectomy. Also, according to Benagiano et al. (2010, Hysterectomy section, para. 2), "most cases of failed vaginal hysterectomy for uterine adenomyosis are due to associated adhesions."

I personally had tremendous success with my laparoscopic hysterectomy. Only the uterus was removed, and all of my abdominal pain completely stopped after the surgery. Recovery from this surgery is longer than some of the other procedures listed here, but it does have a high success rate for relief of adenomyosis symptoms. Obviously, this surgery is not a viable option for those women who still want children.

Laparoscopy – This surgery is done at the hospital, and the patient is put to sleep via general anesthesia. It is typically done as an outpatient procedure. Although not very useful for adenomyosis, this surgery can detect endometriosis, and since both adenomyosis and endometriosis can occur together, this procedure may be an option in treatment. A small incision is made close to the belly button, and the abdomen is filled with gas in order to better view the abdominal organs. A lighted viewing instrument called a laparoscope is placed into the small incision. If areas of endometriosis are found, several more small incisions are made in the lower abdomen, and instruments are guided in to excise or cauterize the endometriosis lesions.

I had one laparoscopy done during my ordeal with adenomyosis. The incisions are small (less than one inch). Recovery took about one week, and I was given some pain medication to take if needed. I don't remember being in tremendous pain – just a little uncomfortable. Be prepared to have some pain in your shoulders. This is due to the remaining gas that they used during surgery to distend the abdomen. The gas rises as you sit up, and you may feel sore in your upper back and shoulders. It feels like the day after a really hard workout at the gym. But the good news is the gas works its way out rather quickly, and this soreness lets up within a few days.

Magnetic resonance-guided focused ultrasound (MRgFUS) – This non-invasive procedure looks promising as the recovery time is shorter and there is a lower risk of complications compared to other procedures. Using magnetic resonance imaging, a beam of energy is sent directly to the adenomyosis lesion and destroys it without injuring any tissue around it. This procedure also looks promising for those women who wish to preserve their fertility. Currently, MRgFUS has been approved for use in the U.S. only for fibroids. The first adenomyosis patient to be treated with MRgFUS had no complications and conceived following the procedure. In addition, the procedure did not affect the pregnancy and delivery of the baby (Taran et al., 2013) According to a study done by Fukunishi et al. (2008), this procedure is effective at destroying most lesions of adenomyosis that are near the serosa of the endometrium. In addition, symptom reduction as well as a lack of serious complications were reported. Kim et al. (2011) evaluated 35 women who had been treated for adenomyosis by MRgFUS, and they concluded the procedure was safe and produced a significant reduction of symptoms. Currently, this procedure looks very promising, but more studies are necessary to ensure its safety.

Myometrial Reduction – This procedure involves removing a large portion of the diseased myometrium by performing a wedge resection with uterine wall reconstruction. This surgery is not advised, however, because of risk of uterine rupture in pregnancy. In addition, the recurrence rate of adenomyosis is high. (Osada et al., 2010). See "Adenomyomectomy" and "Osada procedure".

Osada procedure – This is a modified version of myometrial reduction. After the wedge resection, the uterine wall is reconstructed using a triple-flap method. This method reduces the risk of uterine rupture in future pregnancies. In a study by Osada et al. (2010), 104 women who had severe adenomyosis were treated using this method. After the surgery, all 104 women had a reduction in heavy and painful menstruation. Over fifty percent of the women who wanted to become pregnant were able to carry their pregnancy to term.

Progesterone-releasing IUD (Levonorgestrel) – This kind of IUD is more commonly known as Mirena. The patient lies on her back with her feet in stirrups. Prior to the insertion of the IUD, the physician will do a manual exam to assess the proper placement of the IUD. First, a speculum is used to open up the vagina, and then a tenaculum is inserted to hold the cervix in place. The physician then uses a sound to determine the length of the uterus. This will help in placement of the IUD. The IUD is inserted and opens up into a T-shape once in place. It only takes a couple of minutes to insert an IUD, and some women report pinching or cramping during the procedure. This minor pain should dissipate rather quickly. A couple of strings hang down into the vagina after placement, and the patient is advised to check these strings often to ensure that the IUD is still in place.

In a study by Cho et al. (2008), this type of IUD was found to significantly reduce pain and bleeding, and the reduction of symptoms continued for 36 months. Sheng, Zhang, Zhang, and Lu (2009) were able to obtain similar results in their study and also showed that CA125 levels (a marker for ovarian cancer) dramatically lowered in these women. Mansukhani et al. (2013) report almost 50% of the women were asymptomatic after six months of treatment with a satisfaction rate of 80% (Abstract).

Although the above studies sound promising, I have to address the fact that I have read quite a bit of negative comments about the IUD on online adenomyosis support sites. There have been quite a few women who have reported severe pain after the IUD had been inserted. Many women have stated they went back to their doctor within a week after insertion and demanded to have it removed due to severe pain. Other women have stated they were uncomfortable after it was inserted but pushed through the pain and eventually were pain free. Even though the studies look promising, many times what seems good in theory doesn't work out in real life. I strongly suggest you do your research before you decide to have an IUD implanted. Ask your doctor lots of questions, and even get a second opinion. Adenomyosis causes enough problems, and you certainly don't want to have MORE pain! Another drawback to this IUD is spotting between periods.

Uterine artery embolization (UAE) – During this surgical procedure, a small catheter is inserted into the femoral artery in the groin region. Tiny particles delivered through the catheter block the blood vessels that supply blood to the adenomyotic tissue in the uterus. A study of 20 women by Wang et al. (2010) who had this procedure done revealed disappointing results. Only 15% of these women rated the procedure as satisfactory at 6 months, and 45% of women were dissatisfied. Also, a recent review showed the recurrence rate of adenomyosis after UAE is high (Guo, 2012). According to Bratby & Walker (2009), UAE is helpful in the short-term, but symptoms tend to recur two years after treatment. However, a retrospective study by Siskin, Tublin, Stainken, Dowling, and Dolen (2001) showed the satisfaction rate of UAE at a 12-month follow-up to be 92.3 percent. Postoperative MRI on these patients showed a significant reduction of the size of the junctional zone and the size of the uterus.

Pharmacological treatments

According to a study by Streuli et al. (2014), non-steroidal anti-inflammatory drugs (NSAIDS), progestogens, and gonadotropin-releasing hormone agonists (GnRHas) are the most commonly used medications to treat adenomyosis. However, according to Streuli et al. (2014, Abstract), "There are almost no well-conducted randomized controlled trials on the pharmacological treatment of adenomyosis, and the information collected from published studies is insufficient." The following pharmacological treatments are currently being used to treat adenomyosis:

Aromatase inhibitors – these substances may have some benefit, although studies are few. Several studies have indicated that there may be an abnormal expression of aromatase in endomeriotic and adenomyotic tissue. In a study done by Soysal, Soysal, Ozer, Gul, and Gezgin (2004), the use of aromatase inhibitors in addition to GnRH analogs in women with endometriosis showed promising results as it reduced the risk of recurrence for 24 months.

Progestins – Very few studies have been done on progestins. Dienogest is an oral progestin that had been helpful in the treatment of endometriosis under the name "Visanne". In a study by Hirata et al. (2014), dienogest was found to be an effective treatment for adenomyosis as it reduced pelvic pain, serum CA-125 and CA19-9 levels, and estradiol levels. However, five patients had worsening anemia, a side effect of dienogest.

Continuous birth control pill (BCP) – Low dose BCPs with withdrawal bleeding of about 4 times per year may be helpful. However, no specific studies have been conducted in adenomyosis patients. In addition, since adenomyosis is an estrogen-dependent disorder, this avenue may not be optimal as BCPs contain estrogen.

Vaginal bromocriptine – A study is under way to determine if this treatment would be useful in the treatment of adenomyosis. See "Current Ongoing Studies".

Danazol – Information of the use of danazol in the treatment of adenomyosis is scarce. However, two studies have shown a decrease in painful menstruation. Danazol does have unwanted side effects such as hot flashes.

Gonadotropin-releasing hormone (GnRH) agonists – these substances suppress ovarian function and reduce the amount of estrogen circulating in a woman's body. One study showed a reduction of pelvic pain in women with adenomyosis who were treated with GnRH agonists. There have been a few studies that looked at the use of GnRH agonists along with uterine resection surgery in women who wanted to preserve their fertility These studies showed some promise as pregnancies did occur in some cases. However, a few of the pregnancies had complications. One case in the study by Huang, Yang, and Yuan (1998) had threatened preterm labor, and one in a study by Lin, Sun, and Li (1999) was terminated because of threatened uterine rupture.
It needs to be noted that GnRH agonists do induce adverse effects such as hot flashes and a reduction in bone mineral density.

Non-steroidal anti-inflammatory drugs (NSAIDS) – this is a possible treatment available for women who wish to have children. These medications can potentially lessen the amount of blood lost and reduce pain if started two to three days before the start of menstruation.

Natural Alternatives and Exercise

Natural bio-identical and bio-available progesterone cream – Dr. John Lee (2016) coined the name "estrogen dominance". He suggests the use of bio-identical progesterone cream in cases of estrogen dominance, starting on day 8 and ending on day 26 of the menstrual cycle.

Dr Lee's site (www.johnleemd.com, 2016) has loads of information about hormonal imbalance, and it is well worth the time to check it out. He states synthetic progesterone is not the way to go in trying to balance hormone levels. He explains that synthetic hormones act differently in the body as compared to natural hormones and gives the example of how xenoestrogens upset hormonal balance. He also explains that if the progesterone isn't bio-identical, it can't effectively bind to the progesterone receptors. Synthetic (man-made) hormones bind to protein in the liver which makes them water soluble. This is a problem since hormones are lipophilic which means they work in fat, not water. Once they become water soluble, they cannot bind to the progesterone receptors and are readily excreted through the urine. Dr. Lee's progesterone cream is bio-available which means it is not bound to a protein and is free to bind to the progesterone receptors in the body. His cream is certainly top of the line for those who wish to try this for the reduction of adenomyosis symptoms. Improvement may be seen in two months, but it may also take up to six months of use.

Exercise – Even though adenomyosis sufferers feel pretty awful for about two weeks every month, exercise can be incredibly beneficial on those days when you feel decent enough to do so. Did you know exercise increases life expectancy? For every two hours you work out, it adds about one hour on to your life!

Obesity has been linked to an increased production of aromatase which leads to an increased production of estrogen. This is one of the most important reasons for adenomyosis sufferers to try exercise at least three times a week for thirty minutes. Do you have problems trying to exercise three times a week? You don't have to go to a gym. Just make the effort to be a little more active during the day. Here are some helpful tips:

1. Buy a Fitbit®. This has helped me tremendously as it keeps me motivated. The goal for the number of steps per day is 10,000. That sounds like a lot, but it's really not hard to reach that goal, believe it or not. Checking on the number of steps you've taken during the day will keep you motivated to move more, and you can become friends online with other Fitbit® users who can keep you motivated as well.
2. Workout or walk with a friend. Exercising with someone else will keep you accountable.
3. When shopping, park farther away from the store than you usually do. A little extra walking will earn you more steps on your Fitbit®.
4. Take the stairs instead of the elevator. This will also add more steps on your Fitbit®.
5. Try to get your workout/walking done in the morning or early afternoon. Exercising right before bedtime may interrupt your ability to get a good night of sleep.

Exercise also has other benefits that may help adenomyosis sufferers. One great benefit is that it raises serotonin levels and will give you a sense of well-being. Since increased serotonin levels improves mood, it may help those who suffer from depression. It also improves mental health and promotes more restful sleep.

It is important to lift light weights in addition to getting aerobic exercise. As a woman ages and especially near menopause, bone health becomes a concern. One way to prevent osteoporosis is by lifting light weights as a part of your exercise regime. Lifting weights, even light ones, slows the loss of bone density.

And finally, there are other benefits of exercise that are just good for overall health. Exercise boosts HDL (good cholesterol) and reduces LDL (bad cholesterol). This will help keep your heart and cardiovascular system healthy. Exercise also reduces the risk of type-2 diabetes and some forms of cancer. So, when you are feeling strong enough, try and exercise. If you can get at least thirty minutes of exercise three times per week, you should feel better, and your body may become better equipped to deal with adenomyosis.

Chapter 11 - Infertility and Adenomyosis

Infertility has been reported in women with adenomyosis although no epidemiological studies have been done to confirm this finding. De Souza, Brosens, Schwieso, Paraschos, and Winston (1995) report in women with painful and heavy periods who also had problems with infertility had a 54 percent incidence of JZ hyperplasia. Seventy percent of these women never had children. In animal experiments, baboons with adenomyosis have also had infertility problems and endometriosis (Campo et al., 2012). Studies have also shown an increase in the risk of pre-term delivery in women with both adenomyosis and endometriosis. This could possibly be due to failure of deep implantation of the placenta due to JZ thickening.

Campo et al. (2012) report in women who undergo in vitro fertilization (IVF), evaluation of the junctional zone thickness via MRI is the best way to predict implantation failure. This group also noted that if the patient had a JZ thickness of 10 mm or more, treatment with a GnRH analog prior to IVF had an improvement in the success rate of IVF. GnRH decreases the expression of aromatase which, as previously discussed, is overexpressed in women with adenomyosis. Additionally, it is known that effective implantation occurs with minimal JZ contractions. Since hyperperistalsis occurs in women with adenomyosis and endometriosis, this fact could play a significant role in infertility in these cases. Finally, Leyendecker, Kunz, Wildt, Beil, and Deininger (1996) have demonstrated that sperm transport may be compromised. Sadly, one study has shed some disappointing light on the success rate of IVF in women with adenomyosis. Vercellini et al. (2014) performed a meta-analysis of published data on this subject and found that "adenomyosis appears to impact negatively on IVF/ICSI outcome owing to reduced likelihood of clinical pregnancy and implantation and increased risk of early pregnancy loss" (Abstract).

An issue that may affect fertility in women with adenomyosis is the dysregulation of several proteins. Liu, Duan, and Wang (2013) used mass spectrometry and found 12 areas where proteins were dysregulated in adenomyosis. These abnormal protein expressions may cause the loss of normal rhythmic contractions in the JZ. This may play a role in proper sperm transport needed for a successful pregnancy. In addition, a study by Yen et al. (2006), showed some implantation markers that are seen during normal implantation of the embryo in the uterus are decreased in women with adenomyosis. They suggest this may be a factor in a decrease in implantation rate.

Another factor may involve the presence of excessive free radicals in the uterine environment. Noda et al. (1991) noted a low amount of free radicals is needed to ensure a good environment for the development of the embryo. However, in adenomyosis, it has been shown that the uterus may contain an excessive amount of free radicals, and this may actually damage the fertilized egg (Campo et al., 2012). These free radicals may be attacked by macrophages or T-cells (types of white blood cells), and this may end in an early miscarriage. In conclusion, the adenomyotic uterus appears to be a hostile environment that may significantly contribute to infertility.

Chapter 12 - Could Diet Play a Role?

Studies have shown estrogen levels are lower in women who consume a low-fat, high-fiber diet in comparison to women who consumed a high-fat diet full of processed food. This clearly shows that proper diet is of utmost importance in those women who suffer from adenomyosis.

Before I get into specifics, I want to urge you to consider natural and organic food as much as possible, especially foods that are grown locally. Try to purchase foods at local farmer's markets if possible. The reason for this is that many foods sold in supermarkets are loaded with pesticides and herbicides that are known to be endocrine disruptors. This topic will be discussed at length in Chapter 14.

The following list shows the produce sold in supermarkets that contain the HIGHEST amounts of pesticides (Lam, 2015a):

- Apples
- Apricots
- Bell peppers
- Peaches
- Spinach
- Strawberries

The following list shows the produce sold in supermarkets that contain the LEAST amounts of pesticides (Lam, 2015a):

- Avocados
- Bananas
- Broccoli
- Cauliflower
- Corn
- Green onions
- Onions
- Sweet potato

Keep this in mind when referring to the following recommended foods to help treat adenomyosis and estrogen dominance. If you do not have access to natural/organic foods, it is recommended that you wash fresh produce thoroughly before consuming.

B vitamins – These vitamins are known to balance hormone levels and improve liver function. Specifically, they help to break down and eliminate estrogen in the liver. The following list contains foods high in vitamin B complex:

- Avocado
- Bananas
- Beans
- Chicken
- Eggs
- Leafy greens
- Lentils
- Milk
- Nuts
- Pomegranate
- Potatoes
- Salmon
- Tuna
- Turkey
- Whole grain cereals
- Yogurt

Vitamin B6 – This vitamin helps the body to make serotonin, so it may help with anxiety, depression, and irritability. Excess estrogen competes with vitamin B6, so this vitamin may reduce the levels of estradiol in the body. In 1942, a researcher by the name of Biskind found that a vitamin B deficiency allowed for inefficient metabolization of estrogen in the liver. In addition, studies have found vitamin B6 helps to reduce the symptoms of PMS. This vitamin is also involved in the production of taurine which is necessary for liver health (see Chapter 13). Overall, evidence is fairly strong for use with PMS, menopause, morning sickness, depression, and fibrocystic disease. This vitamin may interact with many medications. Some examples include Dilantin, L-dopa, Luminal (phenobarbital), and Cordarone (WebMD, 2016). Good sources of vitamin B6 include:

- Bananas
- Beans
- Bran
- Brown rice
- Carrots
- Cheese
- Chicken
- Lentils
- Milk
- Russet potatoes
- Salmon (wild)
- Shrimp
- Spinach
- Tuna
- Turkey
- Wheat germ

Vitamin E – This vitamin helps the body to reduce levels of prostaglandins. In addition to being an excellent antioxidant, it is a blood thinner and hormone balancer. Several studies have concluded that vitamin E helps to reduce PMS symptoms. It has also been found to reduce the symptoms of vaginal atrophy and has helped to reduce breast pain. The following foods have high amounts of vitamin E:

- Almonds
- Blueberries
- Olives
- Spinach
- Sunflower seeds

Cruciferous vegetables – These vegetables contain a substance called indole-3-carbinol (I3C) which is known to help detoxify the liver. I3C also helps the body to inactivate estradiol and balance hormone levels. WebMD (2016) reports it is "possibly effective" against cervical dysplasia. However, I3C is known to interact with certain medications, so it is crucial to speak to your physician if you take prescription medications. Avoid excessive consumption in pregnancy. The following is a list of some commonly found cruciferous vegetables:

- Arugula
- Broccoli
- Bok choy
- Brussel sprouts
- Cabbage
- Cauliflower
- Collard greens
- Kale
- Mustard greens
- Radish
- Rutabaga
- Turnip
- Watercress
-

Mushrooms –Mushrooms interfere with the production of aromatase which in turn can lower estrogen levels. Shitake and Portobello are the best to use for this purpose.

Fiber – This nutrient helps to rid the body of excess estrogen by regulating bowel function. By feeding the normal flora in the gastrointestinal tract, fiber helps to metabolize hormones. Fiber also binds to estrogen and helps to eliminate it from the body. An intake of at least 15 grams should be the goal. The following list contains foods high in fiber:

- Fruits, especially prunes, raisins, pears, and raspberries
- Nuts, especially walnuts, almonds, pecans, and peanuts
- Legumes, especially split peas, navy beans, kidney beans and pinto beans
- Whole grains, especially shredded wheat, oatmeal, whole wheat spaghetti, and oatmeal
- Fresh vegetables, especially artichokes, squash, turnip greens, and soybeans
- Rye and/or wheat bread
- Seeds

Sulfur – Foods high in sulfur help to keep the liver functioning properly so it can rid the body of excess estrogen. The following list contains foods high in sulfur:

- Bananas
- Beef
- Chicken
- Chives
- Coconut
- Cruciferous vegetables (see above)
- Egg yolks
- Fish
- Garlic
- Leeks
- Pineapple
- Onions
- Watermelon

Magnesium - Foods high in magnesium may help increase progesterone production. Magnesium may help with bloating, anxiety, insomnia, and breast pain. In fact, taking a calcium and magnesium supplement together at bedtime may aid in more restful sleep. The following list contains foods that are high in magnesium:

- Almonds
- Avocado
- Black beans
- Bran
- Brazil nuts
- Brown rice
- Cashews
- Dark chocolate
- Edamame

- Figs
- Flaxseed
- Kale
- Kidney beans
- Lentils
- Mackerel
- Molasses
- Oatmeal
- Peanuts
- Pumpkin
- Quinoa
- Roast beef
- Sesame seeds
- Spinach
- Squash
- Sunflower seeds
- Swiss chard
- Whole wheat bread

Zinc – This nutrient supports the breakdown and elimination of estrogen by helping to improve liver function. The following foods are high in zinc:

- Baked beans
- Beef
- Cashews
- Chicken
- Crab
- Dark chocolate
- Lamb
- Lobster
- Pine nuts
- Pork
- Pumpkin seeds
- Oysters
- Sunflower seeds
- Wheat germ

Omega-3 fatty acids – These nutrients help the body to balance hormone levels and reduce inflammation. An imbalance of omega-3 to omega-6 fatty acids in the diet has been shown to be a factor in estrogen dominance. A more in-depth discussion of these fatty acids is found in Chapter 17. The following list contains some great sources of omega-3 fatty acids:

- Anchovies
- Canola oil
- Edamame

- Flaxseed
- Halibut
- Herring
- Naturally fed beef and dairy products
- Mackerel
- Olive oil
- Oysters
- Salmon (wild)
- Sardines
- Soybean oil
- Trout
- Tuna
- Walnuts
- Wild rice
- Winter squash

Organic foods – Because of the way they are grown, these foods contain less xenoestrogens (man-made substances that act like estrogen in the body) thereby decreasing the amount of exposure to these dangerous substances.

Resveratrol – This compound contains proanthocyanidins which help block the production of estrogen. Resveratrol is also a type of phytoestrogen called a stilben. A great source is red grapes, but it is also found in peanuts.

Taurine – An essential amino acid, this substance promotes bile circulation and acts as a diuretic. Since it contains sulfur, taurine aids in liver health and toxin removal from the body. Estradiol decreases the amount of taurine formed in the liver, so those with estrogen dominance should ensure that they eat plenty of food that is high in this amino acid. Avoid use in cases of bipolar disorder since taurine is known to interact with lithium. Good food sources include:

- Fish
- Animal meats
- Eggs
- Brewer's yeast

Foods to avoid:

Processed food
Caffeine – Schliep et al. (2012) performed a study in 2012 and found moderate caffeine consumption actually reduced estradiol concentrations in white women. However, intake of caffeinated soda and green tea showed an increase in estradiol concentrations among women of all races. More research is needed to clearly determine the effects of caffeine on estrogen levels.

Coffee – According to Lam (2015b), a study has shown that women who drink 4-5 cups of coffee a day had about 70% more estrogen in their body as compared to women who drank less than one cup per day. He also states that drinking too much coffee may lead to lower production of progesterone and adrenal fatigue.

Refined sugar

Animal meats – Try to eat meats that are naturally fed and hormone-free

Processed dairy products

Alcohol and drugs – Intake of these substances should be reduced or eliminated because of their damaging effects on the liver.

Foods with high amounts of saturated fat

Fried foods

Soft drinks

Chapter 13 - Liver Detoxification

A vital organ, the liver is located in the upper right quadrant of the abdomen and has many functions. It stores vitamins and minerals, makes blood clotting factors, stores glycogen which can be converted into glucose for energy, breaks down nutrients, and is heavily involved in detoxification of toxins that enter the body. These toxins are broken down by Kupffer cells in the liver. This amazing organ also produces bile which is required for the digestion of fats. Of utmost importance in the discussion of adenomyosis is the breakdown and elimination of estrogen. Since estrogen is metabolized in the liver, it is imperative to keep the liver healthy to keep estrogen levels in check. The liver does this in two detoxification pathways – Phase I and Phase II.

In Phase I, the liver converts dangerous toxins into metabolites through the use of enzymes. This process is done through chemical reactions such as oxidation, reduction, and hydrolysis. These processes transform dangerous toxins to a less harmful substance that can be metabolized during Phase II, and this is performed primarily through cytochrome P450. However, in converting these toxins into less harmful substances, free radicals are formed, and these can potentially damage liver cells. The liver produces glutathione which is an antioxidant. As long as the liver is functioning optimally, it produces enough glutathione to neutralize the free radicals produced through the Phase I process. However, if the liver isn't functioning properly, not enough glutathione is produced which may not only lead to liver damage but will also reduce the ability of the liver to break down toxins. The antioxidants that promote proper functioning of this pathway include vitamin A, vitamin B3, vitamin B6, vitamin B12, vitamin C, vitamin D3, vitamin E, calcium, bioflavonoids, N-acetyl-cysteine, quercetin, lipoic acid, grape seed extract, and milk thistle.

In Phase II, the metabolites formed from Phase 1 bind to another substance (cysteine, glycine, or sulfur) which neutralizes the toxin. This is done by converting the toxin from a fat-soluble substance to a water-soluble substance. This process is called conjugation. Since they are now water-soluble, these neutralized toxins can be excreted through the bile or urine. Nutrients that aid in the proper functioning of this pathway include taurine, methionine, folic acid, calcium d-glucarate, sulfur, indole-3-carbinol, and N-acetyl-cysteine.

It is necessary to keep both Phase I and Phase II liver detoxification pathways functioning optimally to encourage proper neutralization and elimination of estrogen. It is important to know, however, that there are both "good" estrogen metabolites and "bad" estrogen metabolites The metabolites 2-(OH)-estrone and 2-(OH)-estradiol are considered good metabolites as they are known to be strong antioxidants. The levels of these good estrogens are usually seen in women who exercise moderately and eat a high protein/low fat diet. They also lower LDL (bad) cholesterol and raise HDL (good) cholesterol. The metabolites 16 alpha-(OH)-estrone and 4-(OH)-estrone are considered bad estrogen metabolites. In particular, 16 alpha-(OH) has been shown to be even more powerful than estradiol (Lam, 2015b). These toxic substances have been linked to breast cancer and have a powerful effect on estrogen receptor sites.

As I'm sure you've already concluded, a healthy diet full of vitamins and minerals is necessary in order to keep the liver functioning properly. Supplements may also be a good idea, especially if your diet is lacking in fresh, organic fruits and vegetables.

Bitter herbs have the amazing ability to aid in digestion and have a beneficial effect on the functioning of the liver. Some of these herbs are listed below, and it would be wise to incorporate them into the diet to keep the liver functioning at an optimal level.

Please note: These are my own recommendations based on my own research, and use of these herbs are not guaranteed to help women with adenomyosis. I advise use of an herb based on estrogen/progesterone activity and the results of clinical research. Please consult an herbal expert or your physician before beginning any kind of herbal therapy, especially if taking prescription medication.

Aloe – Not Recommended
Although aloe juice has shown some benefit to liver health, I personally don't recommend its use in adenomyosis since it is known to stimulate the uterus.

Cascara Sagrada – Recommended if needed/Use sparingly
This bitter and astringent herb is well-known for its laxative effects. It is also known for its tonic effects on the liver and gastrointestinal tract. This herb can be quite harsh and can cause cramping, so it should only be used sparingly. Overuse can cause nausea, vomiting, and abdominal pain. The fresh bark is actually poisonous and must be dried for at least a year prior to use. In addition, this herb is contraindicated in pregnancy.

Chia – Recommended
In addition to its high fiber content, chia contains high amounts of omega-3 fatty acids, vitamins, and minerals. Also, this wonderful food has a very high antioxidant activity level, so it is very beneficial to the liver. In fact, studies have shown significant liver health benefits in rats.

Dandelion – Recommended

This bitter herb has diuretic and laxative effects. It stimulates the liver and has been used to treat cirrhosis, jaundice, hepatitis, and gallbladder disease. Dandelion also improves digestive function.

Lemon balm – Recommended

This herb has both cooling and sedative properties. It improves digestion and relaxes muscle spasms. It has been used to treat indigestion and other digestive issues.

Marshmallow – Recommended

This herb is not the same as the confectionary that is found in grocery stores today. This is an herb that has mucilaginous and expectorant properties that soothe inflamed and irritated tissues, particularly those in the digestive tract.

Milk Thistle – Highly Recommended

This herb is probably the most important of all the herbs when it comes to liver health. Its active constituent, silymarin, is known to protect the liver from toxins and liver damage. It is a bitter, tonic, and diuretic herb that also stimulates bile flow. Milk thistle has a long history of treating poor liver function.

Mullein – Recommended

This bitter herb is also mucilaginous and cooling which is soothing to inflamed and irritated tissues. It also has diuretic and expectorant properties.

Psyllium – Recommended

This fiber supplement is seen quite commonly in drug stores and is touted for its ability to help with constipation. The astringent and cooling properties can be attributed to its active constituent, mucilage. Mucilage swells in the intestine and acts as a laxative. It is also known to absorb toxins in the digestive tract.

Senna – Recommended if needed/Use sparingly

This herb is a laxative and is used to treat constipation. It can be harsh, and it is recommended to be used sparingly. Due to its harshness, it is sometimes given with a carminative herb such as ginger to help with cramping. Overuse can cause nausea, vomiting, and abdominal pain. Its use is contraindicated in pregnancy.

Slippery elm – Recommended

This mucilaginous herb is soothing and helps to draw out toxins from the body. It is useful in a whole host of digestive issues.

In conclusion, a healthy and balanced diet full of fruits, vegetables, lean protein, and healthy fat will help to keep the liver functioning optimally. Use supplements when needed, and try to incorporate some bitter herbs, especially milk thistle. By keeping the liver functioning optimally, it will be better able to process dangerous toxins, especially the dangerous xenoestrogens that may be a contributor to adenomyosis development. A healthy liver will also be able to process estrogen efficiently which will aid in proper elimination, reducing the chance of developing estrogen dominance.

Chapter 14 - All About Xenoestrogens

Xenoestrogens are chemicals that have estrogen-like activity in the human body. They are considered dangerous because they can cause endocrine disruption (altering the function of hormones) which can lead to a whole array of reproductive health problems.

Some scientists and doctors believe that xenoestrogens are harmless to humans and animals because we are routinely exposed to low levels of these chemicals. However, it has been shown that the effects of xenoestrogens are additive, and if we are exposed to low levels of many different ones, it could possibly lead to problems. In addition, according to a study done by Bulayeva and Watson (2004), low levels of these chemicals may be more toxic than previously thought. According to the authors, "These very low effective doses for xenoestrogens demonstrate that many environmental contamination levels previously thought to be subtoxic may very well exert significant signal- and endocrine-disruptive effects, discernable only when the appropriate mechanism is assayed" (Discussion section, para. 3).

The following is a list of some of the most dangerous and recognized xenoestrogens. Many of these chemicals have been banned, but many are still being used today. Also, some of the banned chemicals are still present in the environment since they do not break down easily. Women who suffer from adenomyosis are advised to educate themselves on these chemicals and, although impossible to avoid completely, try to do their best to decrease exposure.

4-methylbenzylidine camphor (4-MBC)

4-MBC is a substance used in sunscreen. In addition to being an endocrine disruptor, it may also play a role in hypothyroidism. Margaret Schlumpf headed a study in Zurich, Switzerland at the Institute of Pharmacology and Toxicolocy (2008) and found 4-MBC applied to rat skin doubled the rate of growth in uterine tissue before puberty. Its use is approved in Europe and Canada, but it is banned in the United States and Japan.

Alkyl phenols (nonylphenols)

These substances have been shown to have clear estrogen activity and should be avoided as much as possible in women who suffer from adenomyosis. They are found in adhesives, carbonless copy paper, detergents, fire retardant materials, fragrances, fuels, lubricants, oil field chemicals, and tires. The use of alkyl phenols is restricted in Europe.

Atrazine

Atrazine is an herbicide that is used on corn, sugarcane, and other crops to control weed growth. It has also been used on golf courses and lawns. In 2014, atrazine was the second most widely used herbicide in the United States, and it is the most commonly detected herbicide in drinking water. Studies have shown it to be an endocrine disruptor; however, the Environmental Protection Agency reports levels are low enough that atrazine probably won't cause reproductive problems. This statement has been criticized, however, and its safety is currently controversial. Tyrone B. Hayes from the University of California at Berkeley (2003) looked at the effect of atrazine on frogs. With increasing exposure to atrazine, some of the frogs began to show both male and female sex organs.

Benzophenone

This substance is used in the printing industry and in sunscreens. It is also used in perfumes and soaps to prevent UV light from damaging their colors and scents.

Bisphenol A (BPA)

BPA is a substance that is used to make epoxy and plastic resins. The major exposure route in humans is through the diet, and it is known to be an endocrine disruptor. BPAs can be found in numerous products such as CDs, DVDs, food and beverage cans, sales receipts (thermal paper), sports equipment, water bottles, and water pipes. In 2013, the Food and Drug Administration reported that BPA is safe at low levels; however, as of 2014, debates persist on its safety. BPA has been banned for use in baby bottles in Canada and Europe. In addition to being an endocrine disruptor, BPAs may play a role in abnormal thyroid function, cancer, diabetes, heart disease, neurological problems, obesity, and reproductive problems.

Butylated hydroxyanisole (BHA)

BHA is an antioxidant used as a food preservative. It can be found in animal food, cosmetics, food, medications, and rubber. The National Institutes of Health report BHA is reasonably anticipated to be carcinogenic due to outcomes of some animal studies; however, in humans, the low intakes don't appear to show an increased risk.

Dichlorobenzene

Dichlorobenzene is a pesticide, deodorant, and disinfectant. It is not easily broken down and can build up in fatty tissues in the human body. It is present in mothballs and is probably carcinogenic.

Dichlorodiphenyltrichloroethane (DDT)

DDT is an insecticide that is classified as "moderately toxic". Its use was banned in 1972. It is a known endocrine disruptor and has been linked to menstrual disorders and other reproductive problems. Studies have also linked it to several types of cancer. A study done by toxicologist Michael Fry at the University of California at Davis (1995) found female cells in the reproductive tracts in male gulls after they were injected with DDT, DDE and methoxychlor. Although banned, DDT can persist in the soil for centuries.

Dieldrin

Dieldrin is an insecticide that was used from the 1950s to the 1970s as an alternative to DDT. It does not easily break down, and it is toxic to both humans and animals. Dieldrin has been linked to reproductive disorders, breast cancer, and Parkinson's disease, and it is banned from use in most parts of the world.

Endosulfan

Endosulfan is an insecticide that treats infestations of whiteflies, aphids, and leafhoppers. It is one of the most toxic pesticides known to man, and its use is being discontinued on a global scale. In addition to being neurotoxic to both humans and animals, it is a clear endocrine disruptor, particularly in males.

Erythrosine (FD&C Red #3)

This substance is a food coloring that is also a possible carcinogen. The Center for Science in the Public Interest has petitioned the U.S. FDA to impose a complete ban of erythrosine, but no action has been taken to date.

Ethinyl estradiol

Ethinyl estradiol is the estrogen component of birth control pills. Through the urine and feces of those who take birth control pills, it is released into the environment as a xenoestrogen.

Hepatachlor

Hepatachlor is an insecticide that can persist in the environment for decades. It is found in breast milk, dairy products, drinking water, fish, and meat. In addition to being a possible carcinogen, hepatachlor may have a negative impact on fertility and the nervous system. Its use is restricted in the United States.

Lindane (gamma-hexachlorocyclohexane)

Lindane is an organochlorine pesticide (OCP) that has been used on humans as a treatment for lice and scabies. β-HCH (β-hexachlorocyclohexane) is a by-product of lindane and has been shown to be a possible endocrine disruptor and carcinogen. Interestingly, a study done in 2013 showed an increased risk of endometriosis in women who were found to have high blood serum levels of β-HCH (Upson et al., 2013). The women in this study with the highest levels of β-HCH were 30 to 70 percent more likely to have endometriosis than the women with the lowest levels of this chemical in their blood serum. In addition, in the same study, the researchers found a slight link between another OCP called Mirex and endometriosis. Mirex was used in the 1960's and 1970's as an insecticide against fire ants. Lindane was banned from use in 2009 except for use as a last resort in the treatment of lice and scabies. However, because Lindane and Mirex are stable and persist in the environment, these two chemicals are still of concern today. The researchers concluded "extensive past use of environmentally persistent OCPs in the United States or present use in other countries may affect the health of reproductive-age women" (Upson et al., 2013, Abstract).

Metalloestrogens

These substances have an affinity for estrogen receptors and are therefore possible endocrine disruptors. They also potentially play a role in breast cancer. The following is a list of metalloestrogens:

- Aluminum
- Antimony
- Arsenite
- Barium
- Cadmium
- Chromium (CRII)
- Cobalt
- Copper
- Lead
- Mercury
- Nickel
- Selenite
- Tin
- Vanadate

Methoxychlor

Methoxychlor is an insecticide that was used as an alternative to DDT. It is a known endocrine disruptor, and it is banned from use.

Parabens

Parabens are preservatives used in cosmetics and other pharmaceutical products such as makeup, moisturizers, shampoos, shaving cream, and toothpaste. They have weak estrogen activity and have been linked to early menarche in young girls.

Pentachlorophenol

Pentachlorophenol is a pesticide and a disinfectant. It is used in wood preservation, paper mills, and masonry. It can be found in leather and rope, and the EPA reports it is probably carcinogenic. Pentachlorophenol is rapidly metabolized, so buildup in the environment is probably not a big issue. Today, this substance is primarily used on utility poles and railroad ties, and it is treated as regulated hazardous waste in the U.S.

Phenosulfonphthalein (Phenol red)

This substance is a red dye that is used in laboratory media as a pH indicator. Phenol red is also found in some home swimming pool test kits. It is a known weak endocrine disruptor.

Polybrominated biphenyls (PBBs)

PBBs are used as flame retardants. These substances don't break down easily in the environment and tend to accumulate. They are found in electrical products, plastic foam, rugs, textiles, and upholstery. PBBs are possible menstruation disruptors. In one study, young girls who were exposed to high levels of PBBs were shown to start menstruating at an earlier age.

Polychlorinated biphenyls (PCBs)

PCBs are used in coolant fluids to help reduce the chance of fire in electrical fields. These substances do not readily decompose and can therefore build up in the environment. They are carcinogenic and have been banned from use since 1979. They were found in carbonless copy paper, caulk, cements, hydraulic fluids, lubricating oils, paints, and pesticides. Also, they are known endocrine and nervous system disruptors. PCBs imitate and inhibit estradiol in the human body which may lead to all kinds of menstrual and reproductive disorders and cancers.

Propyl gallate

This substance is an antioxidant added to foods as a preservative. It is also used in adhesives, animal food, bath products, cosmetics, hair care products, lubricants, sunscreen and toothpaste. It is a known estrogen antagonist.

Phthalates

Phthalates are substances that are added to plastic to increase flexibility (plasticizers). DEHP, or di(2-ethylhexyl) phthalate, is one example that can leach from hospital IV bags. The FDA has warned prolonged treatment with IV fluid bags may affect testicular development in young males. Phthalates have been shown to be endocrine disruptors in studies in rats. According to a study by Moore, Rudy, Lin, Ko, and Peterson (2001), the phthalate DEHP affects the development of the male reproductive system in rats and caused severe reproductive toxicity in five out of eight litters. Phthalates can be found in adhesives, building supplies, butter, caulk, children's toys, detergents, eye shadow, food containers, floor tiles, hair spray, meats, medication, milk, nail polish, nutritional supplements, packaging materials, paints, printing ink, shower curtains, and upholstery. Europe and the United States have restricted the use of phthalates in children's toys.

Sodium lauryl sulfate

This substance is a surfactant that is quite often contaminated with the dangerous chemical 1,4-dioxane. The FDA recommends limits on 1,4-dioxane content in cosmetics but has not established a specific limit. Sodium lauryl sulfate can be found in bubble baths, cleaning products, some food products, laundry detergents, pesticides, shampoo, shaving cream, and toothpaste.

Triclosan

This is an antibacterial and antifungal agent that is often used in hospitals, and it is especially useful when dealing with patients with MRSA (methicillin-resistant staphylococcus aureus). Its safety is under review in both the U.S. and Canada. Triclosan can be found in deodorants, detergents, hospital scrubs, mouthwash, shampoos, soaps, and toothpaste.

So How Can I Reduce My Exposure?

It is virtually impossible to completely eliminate exposure to xenoestrogens. Every day, we are exposed to them the moment we walk out the front door. The goal should be to minimize exposure. Although some exposure to xenoestrogens is out of our control, some are within our control. The following list contains suggestions on ways to minimize your exposure to these dangerous endocrine disruptors.

Note: This is not a comprehensive list. There are other good products out there that contain low or no xenoestrogens. If the products below don't work for you, there may be others that will - just check the labels.

- Do not store or heat any food in a plastic container. All food should be stored and/or heated in glass or ceramic containers.
- Avoid using plastic wrap to store food.
- Use unbleached paper products.
- Use natural fragrances such as pure essential oils. The following company produces high quality essential oils:
    DoTerra®
- Use all natural laundry detergents. The following are some of the top rated products:
    1. Seventh Generation® Natural Powder Laundry Detergent – Real Citrus and Wild Lavender
    2. Seventh Generation® Natural Powder Laundry Detergent – White Flower and Bergamot Citrus
    3. Seventh Generation® Natural Laundry Detergent, Free and Clear
    4. Sun and Earth 2x Concentrated Laundry Detergent – Lavender or Unscented
    5. Martha Stewart® Clean Laundry Detergent
    6. Green Shield® Organic Laundry Detergent, Free and Clear
    7. Nature Clean® Laundry Detergent, Unscented
    8. The Honest Company® Honest 4 in 1 laundry Pods, Free and Clear
- Use all natural dish detergent. The following are some good options:
    1. Whole Foods Market® Liquid Dish Soap, Mandarin Ginger
    2. Eco-Me® Dish Soap
    3. Seventh Generation® Automatic Dishwashing Powder
- Use natural herbicides and pesticides. There are many ways to naturally control pests. The following options are easy to prepare:
    1. 1 cup salt/1-gallon vinegar. Mix and put in a spray bottle.
    2. Fill a spray bottle half full with vinegar and finish filling it with all natural liquid soap.
    3. Sprinkle diatomaceous earth around plants.
    4. Sprinkle small amount of eucalyptus oil around plants.
    5. Use onion, garlic, or cayenne pepper for pest control.
    6. For ants, use 1 tbsp. peppermint essential oil in 1 liter of water and put in spray bottle. Another option is to put 5-10 drops of any citrus essential oil and 1 tsp. cayenne pepper in 1 quart of water. Put in spray bottle.

7. Use ½ tsp. neem, ½ tsp. natural liquid soap, fill to one gallon with water and put into a spray bottle.
- Use all natural cleaning products. Try the following natural options:
    1. Seventh Generation® Toilet Bowl Cleaner
    2. Green Shield® Organic Toilet Bowl Cleaner
    3. Seventh Generation® Natural Tub and Tile Cleaner – Emerald Cypress and Fir
    4. Biokleen® Carpet and Rug Shampoo
    5. Earth Friendly Products® Concentrated Carpet Shampoo with Bergamot and Sage
    6. The Honest Company® products
- Only buy grass fed organic meats that say "hormone free".
- Avoid salmon that has been farm-raised as it contains high levels of PCBs. Look for "wild" salmon.
- Buy organic fruits and vegetables. If you do buy non-organic fruits and vegetables, peel them before eating.
- Restrict intake of dairy products.
- Use a high quality water filter.
- Avoid birth control pills. Use a condom (without a spermicide) or an IUD instead.
- Use bioidentical hormones to treat hormonal imbalances.
- Use all natural baby products. The following are some good options:
    1. Babyganics® Foaming Dish and Bottle Soap
    2. The Honest Company® products
    3. Baby Earth® products
- Use natural cosmetics. Try out some of the following natural products:
    1. Bare Minerals® products
    2. Origins® products
    3. Devita® products
    4. Earth's Beauty® products
    5. Lavera® products
    6. Ecco Bella® products
    7. Bella Floria® products
    8. Burt's Bees® tinted lip balm
    9. Physicians Formula® products
    10. It Cosmetics®
- Use natural lotions and moisturizers. Try out some of the following natural products:
    1. 100% Pure® products
    2. Bella Floria® products
    3. Aroma Bella® Skin Care
    4. Nature's Gate® Face Moisturizer
- Use natural toothpaste. The following are some top-rated products:
    1. Toms of Maine® Toothpaste
    2. Dr. Ken's® All Natural Maximum Care Toothpaste
    3. Kiss My Face® Triple Action Whitening Toothpaste

- Try to avoid shower curtains – install a glass shower door if possible.
- Use a zinc oxide based sunscreen.
- Try to avoid canned foods. Frozen is better.
- If your home is newly painted or carpeted, make sure there is proper ventilation.
- Avoid plastic water bottles.
- Use natural soaps. The following are some good options:
    1. Dr. Bronner's® 18-in-1 Hemp Pure Castile Soap or any Castile soap
    2. Ballard Organics® All Purpose Concentrated Liquid Soap – Jasmine/Bergamot
    3. The Honest Company® products
- Use all natural shampoos and conditioners. The following are some good products to try out:
    1. L'oreal Paris® Ever Pure Moisture Shampoo
    2. Avalon Organics® Revitalizing Peppermint Shampoo
    3. Burt's Bees® Super Shiny Grapefruit and Sugar Beet Shampoo
    4. TIGI S-Factor® Color Savvy Shampoo
    5. Aveda® Shampure Shampoo
    6. The Honest Company® products
- I personally try to avoid the fertilizer/pesticide area in home improvement stores. As soon as I get near the area, I can smell those products. If I can smell them, I feel like I am probably being exposed to them.

In conclusion, xenoestrogens are known endocrine disruptors that have been shown many times to affect the functioning of the reproductive tract in both males and females. Although not all scientists and doctors agree on the toxicity of these substances, it would be a good idea to reduce exposure as much as possible, especially in women who suffer from adenomyosis. According to Slomczynska in an article in the Polish Journal of Veterinary Science (2008), "There is a need for the studies on all potential xenoestrogens to describe tissue specific activities, and via which pathways in those tissues these compounds wither disrupt or mimic hormone action" (Abstract).

Chapter 15 - Can Phytoestrogens Help?

In researching phytoestrogens and their bioactivity in preparation for this book, I realized that this subject is far more complicated than I first thought. In this chapter, I will attempt to clarify as much as possible how phytoestrogens work in the body and discuss which phytoestrogens may help with adenomyosis.

The role of phytoestrogens in women with adenomyosis and estrogen dominance is confusing, to say the least. There is some disagreement within the natural health care and medical field as to whether or not phytoestrogens increase estrogen levels or help to combat estrogen dominance. Before I go any further, it is important to understand the basics on how different types of estrogen exert their influence in the human body.

In a woman's body, many different tissues have estrogen receptors. Think of it as a couple of puzzle pieces. When estrogen becomes available, it will fit into one of these receptor sites (puzzle slots). Once in place, through a series of chemical reactions, estrogen will begin to exert its influence on the ovaries, uterus, or other organs that are susceptible to estrogen's influence.

There are many different types of estrogen. The three that are discussed here are endogenous estrogen, xenoestrogens, and phytoestrogens. Endogenous estrogen is made in a woman's body and is produced specifically for the proper functioning of the reproductive tract. Xenoestrogens, as discussed previously, are dangerous, man-made substances that act like estrogens in the body and are many times more powerful than human estrogen. They should be avoided at all costs. In general, most phytoestrogens are found in foods and plants and are much weaker than endogenous estrogen.

Although not all natural health care practitioners are in agreement, many believe that a diet high in phytoestrogens will improve conditions associated with estrogen dominance. The theory is that phytoestrogens will bind up the estrogen receptor sites. Therefore, if a woman is exposed to excess amounts of estradiol and/or xenoestrogens, there would be very little to bind to, so these dangerous estrogens would not be activated within the body. Also, since phytoestrogens are much weaker, the estrogenic effect in a woman's body would be much weaker, thereby reducing the risk of estrogen dominance.

Some studies confirm this theory. A study by Rebbeck et al. (2007) showed the use of black cohosh in women with breast cancer may have a protective effect. Black cohosh has been used for many years to treat menopausal symptoms, and it is reported to have anti-estrogenic effects. The authors of this study caution it is not clear exactly how black cohosh works, and its activity may not actually be associated with hormonal status. In addition, Bacciottini et al. (2007) report genistein has one third of the potency when it binds to ERα and one thousandth of the potency when it binds to ERβ as compared to endogenous estrogen. Two estrogen receptor sites are currently known – ERα and ERβ. Phytoestrogens bind to both, but prefer to bind to ERβ (Bacciottini et al., 2007).

Some practitioners do not agree, however. Some advise avoiding foods that contain phytoestrogens, such as soy, in cases of estrogen dominance. Soy contains the highest level of isoflavones in any food source, and these isoflavones are the strongest form of phytoestrogens known. Patisaul & Jefferson (2010, Section 7.4, para. 2) report the phytoestrogen in soy, genistein, "alters ovarian differentiation, reduces fertility and causes uterine cancer later in life" in mice studies. They also report genistein alters ovarian function in mice. However, they conclude in their report that "Moderation is likely key and the incorporation of real foods, as opposed to supplements or processed foods to which soy protein is added, is probably essential for maximizing health benefits." (Section 9, para. 2).

It is important to understand each phytoestrogen works differently. Recently, some studies have been done that show some phytoestrogens are as potent as estradiol. Some help with menopausal symptoms by raising estrogen levels while others, such as black cohosh, are anti-estrogenic.

Zava, Dolbaum, and Blen (1998) performed a very detailed study of some of the most common herbs and their interactions with estrogen and progesterone receptors by identifying them as agonists or antagonists. An agonist refers to a substance that binds with a receptor and activates it, and an antagonist refers to a substance that binds to the receptor without exhibiting a biological response. In the case of adenomyosis, herbs that are estrogen antagonists and progesterone agonists are optimal. It is inadvisable to use strong estrogen agonists due to the possibility of worsening estrogen dominance.

Much more research needs to be done to fully understand how phytoestrogens work in the human body. Many factors have not been addressed such as absorption, bioavailability once the food/herb has been ingested, and the effects and interactions of other substances in the food/herb. In addition, the way the herb acts in these studies (in vitro) may not be the way the food/herb actually acts in the human body (in vivo).

Keep in mind since most phytoestrogens are weak estrogens, you would likely have to consume a very large amount of them to put yourself into an estrogen dominant condition. According to Seidl and Stewart (1998, Results section, para. 5), "the relative potency of phytoestrogens is, at most, only 2% that of estradiol." Also, they report consumption of phytoestrogens are considered safe. In my opinion, I do believe a diet high in phytoestrogens will help protect a woman from the harmful effects of xenoestrogens. But the decision really is up to the patient. Again, consultation with a physician or natural health care expert is of utmost importance. Hormone testing is also advisable.

The following foods are known to be good sources of phytoestrogens:

- Almonds
- Apples
- Barley
- Beans
- Berries
- Cabbage
- Carrots
- Flaxseed
- Garlic
- Grapes
- Lentils
- Multigrain bread
- Oats
- Onion
- Pears
- Pistachios
- Plums
- Pomegranate
- Rice
- Rye bread
- Sesame seeds
- Spinach
- Sprouts
- Sunflower seeds
- Tea
- Wheat
- Wine
- Yams

Chapter 16 - Supplement Review and Recommendations for Adenomyosis

As you learned in the previous chapter, the subject of phytoestrogens can be very confusing. The supplements below are considered phytoestrogens. I have researched each of the herbs/supplements and have found that although a lot of them are known to "balance hormones", they do so in different ways. Some are estrogen agonists, some are progesterone agonists, and some are both estrogen and progesterone agonists. It is important to note these differences. Some of the "hormone balancers" raise estrogen levels and may help women who are low in estrogen (during menopause). Others raise progesterone levels which in theory should help women with endometriosis and adenomyosis. For adenomyosis patients (and endometriosis, for that matter), the herbs used should be known progesterone agonists. Estrogen agonists may possibly increase estrogen levels, so adenomyosis sufferers should be wary of these types of herbal supplements.

Please note: These are my own recommendations based on my own research, and successful use of these herbs are not guaranteed to help women with adenomyosis. I advise use of an herb based on estrogen/progesterone activity and the results of clinical research. Please consult an herbal expert or your physician before beginning any kind of herbal therapy.

Anise – Caution/Not recommended

This herb has historically been used to treat menstrual pain, ease childbirth, increase milk flow, and increase sex drive. WebMD (2016) reports anise is possibly effective for menstrual discomfort. However, WebMD (2016) also states anise has estrogen-like activity and is not recommended in women with hormone-sensitive conditions. For this reason, I do not recommend the use of anise in women with adenomyosis.

Cautions: Interacts with birth control pills, estrogen drugs, and Tamoxifen.

Black Cohosh – Recommended

A member of the buttercup family, this wonderful herb has been used extensively by the North American Indians. It has a long history of use for premenstrual syndrome and menstrual cramping, and it may also be helpful with menopause symptoms such as irritability, hot flashes, and vaginal dryness.

Although studies on black cohosh have been conflicting, most seem to point to very little or no estrogenic activity. Liske, Hanggi, and Henneicke-von Zepelin (2002) report women who took Remifemin tablets (which contain black cohosh extracts) for 6 months showed no changes in LH, FSH, prolactin or estradiol levels. Liu, Burdette, and Xu (2001) showed black cohosh had no activity in estrogen receptor binding in S30 (breast cancer) and Ishikawa (endometrial) cells. Zava et al. (1998) report black cohosh has little estrogenic bioactivity, and Seidl and Stewart (1998, Table 2) state there is "no evidence of estrogenic effect in study of uterine growth in immature mice…".

Cautions: Excessive use may cause headaches and gastrointestinal upset. Avoid use during pregnancy or in cases of breast cancer or liver disorders. This herb may interfere with birth control pills.

Chasteberry – see Vitex

Damiana - Recommended
Known for its aphrodisiac properties, this herb may help with anxiety, depression, hot flashes, and night sweats. It may inhibit aromatase which is needed to convert androgens to estrogen. A 1998 study found that this herb had anti-estrogenic activity, and, according to Zava et al. (1998), this herb is one of the six highest progesterone-binding herbs. It has also been noted that this herb may contain compounds similar to progesterone. Damiana may interact with other herbs and supplements that alter progesterone levels.

Cautions: Excessive use may cause diarrhea. Avoid use if on diuretics or if diabetic as this herb may affect blood sugar levels.

Dandelion - Recommended
Believe it or not, this little yellow weed is an invaluable herb. Dandelion, also known as "pee in the bed", is a powerful diuretic which could be invaluable if you suffer from severe bloating due to adenomyosis. An additional benefit is this herb will reduce bloating without causing the body to lose large quantities of potassium, an unwanted side effect of diuretic drugs such as Lasix. According to Zhi et al. (2007), this herb may be useful "for the clinical treatment of reproductive hormone-related disturbances" (Abstract).

Cautions: This herb can alter the concentrations of certain antibiotics. Avoid if allergic to chamomile, ragweed, or yarrow. May interact with other diuretics, lithium, and antacids.

Diindolylmethane (DIM) – Possibly helpful
DIM, also known as diindolylmethane, is formed in the body by substances found in cruciferous vegetables. It may act like an estrogen and may increase the levels of good estrogen (Lam, 2015b). Although there is insufficient evidence of its effectiveness, this substance may help prevent breast or uterine cancer and may help reduce the symptoms of PMS. DIM has been used in cases of estrogen dominance; however, the research for this use is lacking.

Cautions: May interact with many different medications including but not limited to Flexeril, theophylline, Inderol, Talwin, and Haldol. Consult a physician before use if taking a prescription medication.

Dong Quai – Recommended
Zava et al. (1998) report that this herb did not inhibit the production of alkaline phosphatase, which means it does not block the activity of progesterone. In addition, this group notes that this herb has very little estrogenic activity. This herb may actually suppress estradiol synthesis since saliva levels in women who take this herb are very low.

Cautions: This herb interacts with blood thinners. Sensitivity to sunlight is increased if taken with St. John's Wort.

European Mistletoe – Caution/Not Recommended
Kim et al. (2014) demonstrated Korean mistletoe water extracts improved symptoms in an estrogen-deficient animal model, so it appears this herb may be an estrogen agonist. However, mistletoe does not block the production of progesterone according to Zava et al. (1998). Marvibaigi, Supriyanto, Amini, Majid, and Jaganathan (2014) showed this herb had some clinical benefit for use in breast cancer, but the action appeared to be through apoptosis and cytotoxicity rather than through an effect on hormonal levels.

Cautions: The mistletoe discussed here refers to European mistletoe. American mistletoe is dangerous and should not be taken internally. Interacts with high blood pressure medication and immunosuppressant drugs.

Evening Primrose Oil – Use with Caution
Evening primrose oil is a natural source of gamma linolenic acid, or GLA. This is a type of omega-6 fatty acid. The American diet is generally high in omega-6 consumption and very low in omega-3 consumption (see Chapter 17). GLA is a precursor to a type of prostaglandin, and prostaglandins increase inflammation and pain. Also there are some reports evening primrose oil can affect estrogen levels, but no carefully conducted clinical trial has been able to confirm these reports. Interestingly, the University of Maryland Medical Center Complementary and Alternative Medicine Guide (2016) states this supplement may help women with endometriosis.

Cautions: interacts with anticoagulant and antiplatelet drugs such as aspirin, ibuprofen, naproxen, heparin, warfarin, Plavix, and Voltaren. Also known to interact with anesthesia and phenothiazines.

False Unicorn – Not Recommended
I do not recommend use of this herb for adenomyosis for two reasons: the herb is endangered, and clinical evidence of its usefulness is severely lacking. Native American women have used it to help prevent miscarriage, and it has also been used to balance hormone levels. However, it is not known for sure how this herb affects hormones.

Fennel – Not Recommended
This herb contains anethole, photoanethole, and dianethole. All three of these substances are believed to have estrogenic properties. Fennel is known to increase milk secretion, increase sex drive, and may impact hormone levels. Not enough is known about the activity of this herb to be able to label it as beneficial or detrimental in women with adenomyosis.

Ginseng – Not Recommended
Ginseng contains high amounts of phytoestrogens. However, this herb may have an estrogenic effect due to the similarity of its active ingredient, ginsenoside, to estrogen (Seidl & Stewart, 1998). Also, there is a reported case of post-menopausal bleeding in a woman who applied a ginseng cream vaginally (Seidl & Stewart, 1998).

Goldenseal – Not Recommended
Zava et al. (1998) report that this herb blocked enzyme production by progesterone, and they labeled goldenseal as an anti-progestin.

Grape Seed Extract - Recommended
Discovered in 1951 by the French scientist Dr. Jacques Masquelier, this amazing supplement has been shown to be a potent aromatase inhibitor. The ability of this supplement to inhibit aromatase may be very beneficial to women who suffer from estrogen dominance. In a study by Kijma, Phung, Hur, Kwok, and Chen (2006), grape seed extract was shown to possibly be a useful treatment in cases of hormone-dependent breast cancer. Grape leaves, especially the leaves of the red grape, have been shown to have astringent qualities, and this might be beneficial in treating heavy menstrual bleeding. In addition, the proanthocyanidins in grape seed extract are powerful antioxidants which can help keep the liver healthy. Although the data is insufficient, grape seed extract may also help in cases of premenstrual syndrome.

Cautions: This supplement can interfere with blood thinners, NSAIDS, and heart medications. Avoid use in bleeding disorders and for at least two weeks prior to having surgery.

Hops – Not Recommended
Zava et al. (1998) report hops has estrogenic effects, and this herb showed significantly higher growth of breast cancer cells when compared to the control.

Licorice – Conflicting Data/Not Recommended
Here, licorice refers to the actual herb. Many licorice products in the United States contain anise which gives it the licorice flavor, but these products do not contain the licorice herb. Substances in licorice have been shown to bind to estrogen receptors. According to Paul Bergner (2001),

glycyrrhiza, a component of licorice, is able to increase progesterone levels in the form of 17-hydroxy-progesterone. In addition, other research has shown that a combination of licorice and peony may reduce prolactin levels. Licorice has been used to treat polycystic ovarian syndrome although the research is lacking regarding its effectiveness.

Even so, licorice may have some estrogenic activity, and WebMD.com (2016) recommends that it not be used in hormone-sensitive conditions. Also, according to Zava et al. (1998), this herb is one of the six highest estrogen-receptor binding herbs. This group also notes cell growth in breast cancer cell lines showed significantly higher growth when compared to the control cell line. They list this herb as an anti-progestin since it blocked the induction of alkaline phosphatase.

Melatonin - Recommended

This hormone is produced in the pineal gland and is important in modulating our circadian rhythms. It is also a free radical scavenger, helps with the proper functioning of the immune system, and plays an important role in the regulation of sex hormones. Recent studies have shown this hormone may reduce binding to estrogen receptors while it increases binding to progesterone receptors. A study by Rato et al. (1999) showed melatonin interfered with the activation of an estrogen receptor by estradiol. Abd-Allah, El-Sayed, Abdel-Wahab, and Hamada (2003) showed a 59 percent reduction of estrogen receptors in rats that were treated with melatonin. In addition, this same group showed an increase in progesterone receptors of 53 percent in these same rats.

Cautions: Interacts with sedatives, birth control pills, diabetic medications, caffeine, and antiplatelet/anticoagulant drugs such as aspirin, ibuprofen, naproxen, Plavix, and Voltaren.

Milk Thistle - Recommended

This amazing herb has been known for thousands of years to protect and nourish the liver. Silymarin is the active constituent of the plant, and this substance protects the liver from damage by toxins several ways. First of all, it is a strong antioxidant, and it has been shown to be more effective than both vitamin C and vitamin E. It also helps to prevent the depletion of glutathione which is needed for the proper functioning of the liver. Silymarin has been repeatedly shown to be beneficial in treating cirrhosis and hepatitis. Since estrogen is processed in the liver, it is vital to keep the liver healthy, so the addition of this herb to the diet of adenomyosis sufferers is an excellent idea!

Cautions: May interfere with the effectiveness of birth control pills. May cause vomiting and diarrhea if consumed in excess. May interfere with acetaminophen, general anesthesia, nitrous oxide, chemotherapy drugs, methotrexate, Lovastatin, Pravastatin, Haloperidol, Metronidazole, Paclitaxel, Cisplantin, Tacrine, and Clofibrate.

Motherwort – Caution/Conflicting Data

This herb has been used for amenorrhea. Tao et al. (2009) state Chinese motherwort ethanol extract may inhibit the proliferation of breast cancer cells. This group also states motherwort "markedly suppressed the development of uterine adenomyosis and mammary cancers in mice" (Abstract). However, Zava et al. (1998) report that this herb has possible estrogenic effects, and growth of breast cancer cells were significantly higher as compared to control. Due to the conflicting data on this herb, I caution its use in adenomyosis.

N-acetyl-cysteine (NAC) - Recommended

NAC is an excellent antioxidant and chelator of heavy metals. It is an excellent supplement as it aids in optimum liver function. It is derived from the amino acid cysteine and contains a good amount of sulfur.

Cautions: Interacts with nitroglycerin and activated charcoal.

Nutmeg – Not Recommended

Zava et al. (1998) report that this herb blocked enzyme induction by progesterone, thus labeling it as an anti-progestin.

Oregano – Recommended

According to Zava et al. (1998), oregano is one of the six highest progesterone binding herbs. In addition, the volatile oils in oregano help to detoxify the liver.

Cautions: Since this herb may lower blood sugar levels, use with caution in cases of diabetes. Oregano may also interact with lithium.

Pennyroyal – Not Recommended

Zava et al. (1998) report that this herb blocked enzyme induction by progesterone, thus labeling it as an anti-progestin.

Quercetin - Recommended

Quercetin is a plant flavonoid and a strong aromatase inhibitor. A study done by van der Woude et al. (2005) showed that quercetin exerts phytoestrogen-like activity. The group states "the results point at the relatively high capacity of quercetin to stimulate supposed 'beneficial' [estrogen receptor] beta responses as compared to the stimulation of [estrogen receptor] alpha, the receptor possibly involved in adverse cell proliferative effects" (Abstract). Quercetin is found in red wine, green tea, onions, berries, and apples. It works best when taken with Vitamin C.

Cautions: Excessive use can cause headaches and tingling in the arms and legs. Consultation with a physician is imperative if taking prescription medications as there are many interactions. Some examples include Cipro, cyclosporine, Zantac, Tagamet, and Allegra.

Red Clover – Not recommended

The high content of isoflavones in red clover are converted into phytoestrogens in the body. Although this would seem like a good thing, the evidence of its usefulness is scarce, and there is a warning to avoid this particular herb in cases of hormone-sensitive disorders. In fact, according to Zava et al. (1998), it is one of the six highest estrogen-receptor binding herbs but it is also listed as one of the six highest progesterone-binding herbs. Zava et al. (1998) also note that the potency of red clover is similar to estradiol. In addition, this herb is known to interact with a whole host of medications including but not limited to estrogens, birth control pills, and tamoxifen.

Rosemary – Recommended

According to the Cleveland Clinic (2016), rosemary may lower estrogen levels. This herb is also anti-inflammatory, and its volatile oils aid in liver detoxification.

Cautions: Since rosemary may be toxic to embryos (Cleveland Clinic, 2016), avoid use during pregnancy or if trying to become pregnant. May interact with lithium.

Royal Jelly – Possibly Useful

This nutritious supplement is made from bees. The major constituent is water (67%), but it also contains many nutrients such as protein, sugars, fatty acids, minerals, enzymes, vitamin B5, vitamin B6, and a little bit of vitamin C. It has been used for PMS, insomnia, menopause, and liver disease, and it has been reported to decrease inflammation and nourish the endocrine system. According to Hiroyuki et al (2012), this supplement appears to increase testosterone levels in men and also appears to have no effect on the conversion of aromatase in humans. Caffeic acid phenethyl ester (CAPE) is a substance that is found in bee propolis. Jung et al. studied CAPE in 2010 and found that it had binding affinity to ERβ. Also, CAPE did not increase the growth of MCF-7 estrogen receptor-positive breast cancer cells, and it did not increase the uterine weight.

Cautions: There is a risk of allergic reaction with this supplement. There have been reports of asthma, hives, and even anaphylaxis, so use with caution especially if you have a history of allergies. Avoid use if taking warfarin or if pregnant.

SAMe – Recommended
Also known as s-adenosyl methionine, this substance is made in the body as a result of a reaction between methionine and ATP. Methionine must be supplied through the diet as it cannot be made by the body. SAMe is an excellent source of sulfur and helps to convert estradiol (E2) into the less harmful estriol (E3). SAMe has been used for PMS and premenstrual dysphoric disorder (PMDD), a more severe form of PMS. It has also been used to help with depression and may even be useful in liver disease. SAMe is an anti-inflammatory and used to relieve pain. An interesting study by Frezza, Tritapepe, Pozzato, and Di Padova (1988) looked at the use of SAMe in women who had a past history of liver disease called intrahepatic cholestasis of pregnancy (ICP). These women have an increased sensitivity to estrogen. They concluded "The data support the belief that SAMe acts as a physiological antidote against estrogen hepatobiliary toxicity in susceptible women" (Abstract).

Cautions: Do not use if you have bipolar disorder or Parkinson's disease. May react with dextromethorphan, antidepressants (including MAOIs), St. John's Wort, levodopa, Demerol, Talwin, and Ultram. Since so little evidence is available for this supplement, it is highly advised to consult a physician before use. It is advised to take folic acid and vitamin B6 with this supplement as excessive intake of methionine alone has been linked to stroke and heart disease.

Soy – Recommended in Moderation
Soy is a very complicated topic when it comes to its effects on hormonal levels. There are many misconceptions about soy. The interest in soy and hormone levels came as a result of the fact that Asian women had a much lower risk of breast cancer than women in the U.S. In fact, women in the East Asia eat about ten times more soy than women in the U.S., but their hormone-positive breast cancer rates are far lower. This topic was discussed on the Dr. Oz show (2015) as they tried to clear up some misconceptions. They stated that soy can reduce breast cancer risk if eaten on a regular basis. However, in women who already have breast cancer, this benefit is questionable, so soy consumption is cautioned. They also state that the best types of soy are edamame, tofu and fermented soy products. Kurzer (2002, Abstract) states "soy and isoflavone consumption does not seem to affect endometrium in pre-menopausal women…". Additionally, Barrett (2006) states that soy inhibits aromatase and inhibits angiogenesis. She also states a study showed that genistein, a component of soy, may inhibit the growth of breast cancer cells.

In contrast, some animal studies have shown consumption of large amounts of soy reduced fertility and triggered premature puberty in animal studies. A study done by Jefferson, Padilla-Banks, and Newbold (2007) report mice that were given genistein neonatally showed altered ovarian function and reduced fertility. Zava et al. (1998) lists soy as one of the six most potent estrogen-binding products. However, they also note that genistein in soy suppresses estradiol synthesis.

Cautions: Interacts with MAOI antidepressants, antibiotics, warfarin, Tamoxifen, and estrogen drugs.

Thyme – Caution/Use in Small Amounts
Zava et al. (1998) reports this herb as one of the six highest estrogen-receptor binding herbs, but it is also listed as one of the six highest progesterone-binding herbs. The volatile oils in thyme aid in liver detoxification. WebMD (2016) says to avoid use of this herb in hormone-sensitive conditions such as endometriosis. Since it is one of the six highest progesterone binding herbs, it might be safe to use this herb in small amounts in women with adenomyosis.

Cautions: Interacts with anticoagulants and antiplatelet drugs such as aspirin, ibuprofen, naproxen, Plavix, and Voltaren.

Turmeric – Caution/Not Enough Evidence
Turmeric is an excellent anti-inflammatory herb. Its active ingredient, curcumin, is known to be a powerful antioxidant. WebMD (2016) reports even though curcumin may act like estrogen in the body, studies have shown it may reduce the action of estrogen in hormone-sensitive cancer cells. However, evidence is limited, so its use is cautioned.

Cautions: May interact with antiplatelet or anticoagulant drugs such as aspirin, ibuprofen, naproxen, Plavix, and Voltaren. Use with caution in gallbladder disease, diabetes, gastroesophageal reflux disease, and bleeding disorders.

Vitex (Chasteberry) - Recommended
Vitex is also known as "the woman's herb" and is known for its hormone-balancing effects. It influences the pituitary gland to produce luteinizing hormone which, in turn, signals the ovaries to produce progesterone. Vitex may also lower prolactin levels. It has been used to treat fibrocystic disease, abnormal menstrual bleeding, PMS, PMDD, polycystic ovarian syndrome, uterine fibroids, miscarriage, low progesterone levels, menopausal symptoms, and infertility. In a 1988 study, researchers looked into the effects of this herb in women with luteal phase defect (low progesterone levels). Forty-five women with this defect took vitex once a day for 3 months, and progesterone levels returned to normal in 25 of the women (WholeHealthMD.com, 2005). This group also states this herb may help to relieve endometriosis pain. According to Seidl and Stewart (1998), this herb is found to be effective in cases of hyperprolactinemia. In addition, Vitex

appears to be comparable in effectiveness to Prozac in the treatment of PMDD.

Cautions: Vitex should not be used in those with Parkinson's disease, those who have schizophrenia, women who are undergoing in vitro fertilization, or women who are pregnant. May interact with birth control pills, estrogens, medication for Parkinson's disease, antipsychotic medications, and Reglan. Avoid if using bromocriptine.

Wild Yam – Not Useful

Diosgenin, a phytoestrogen found in wild yam, was used to make the contraceptive pill until 1970. An organic chemist found that he could produce progesterone from wild yam in 1943. However, according to Zava et al. (1998), saliva tests on women using products containing diosgenin showed very low levels of progesterone. This result confirms recent reports diosgenin is not converted into progesterone in the human body. The conversion apparently only takes place in the lab through a chemical process.

Yucca – Not Recommended

Zava et al. (1998) found yucca had possible estrogenic effects that were equivalent to estradiol. Interestingly, it did not block progesterone either. However, since its estrogenic effects are so potent, I do not recommend this herb for use in women with adenomyosis.

Chapter 17 - Omega-3 Fatty Acids May Offer Some Hope

Omega-3 fatty acids fall into the category of essential fatty acids (EFAs). In order to completely understand the role of omega-3 fatty acids in the human body, it is important to understand the difference between saturated and unsaturated fats.

Fats, also called lipids, are made from hydrogen, carbon, and oxygen. Ninety-five percent of fats are in the form of triglycerides while the other five percent are made up of phospholipids and sterols. One type of sterol is cholesterol. Fats are also divided into two kinds: saturated and unsaturated. In a saturated fat, every carbon is linked to a hydrogen atom. In an unsaturated fat, the carbons are not completely saturated with hydrogen atoms. This means some of the carbon atoms contain double bonds. A monounsaturated fat contains one double bond. Examples are olive, peanut, and canola oil. Polyunsaturated fats have more than one double bond. Omega-3 and omega-6 fatty acids are both polyunsaturated fatty acids. Examples include fish oil, soybean oil, and sunflower oil.

Over the last ten to twenty years, there has been a lot of talk about trans fats. These types of fats are manufactured fats that are not in their natural form. They are manufactured through a process called hydrogenation. This process aids in the shelf life of products since fats in their natural form tend to turn rancid rather quickly. However, research has shown that these unnatural trans fats are extremely unhealthy. It is advised to avoid them at all costs.

Essential fatty acids have many benefits. They regulate the metabolism of cholesterol and maintain the integrity of cell membranes by keeping them fluid and flexible. This allows for efficient exchange of nutrient into and out of the cell. They are also precursors to prostaglandins, thromboxanes, leukotrienes, and lipoxins which are vital hormones involved in the inflammatory process. In addition, omega-3 fatty acids in particular have been shown to help the body balance hormone levels. An imbalance of omega-3 to omega-6 fatty acids in the diet appears to be a factor in estrogen dominance.

Essential fatty acids are called "essential" because they cannot be made in the body and must come from the diet. The two essential fatty acids are linoleic acid (LA) and alpha linolenic acid (LNA). LA is an omega-6 fatty acid, and LNA is an omega-3 fatty acid.

LA is converted in the body to other omega-6 fatty acids including gamma linoleic acid (GLA) and arachidonic acid (AA). LNA is converted in the body to other omega-3 fatty acids which include docohexanoic acid (DHA) and eisosapentenoic acid (EPA). Both EPA and DHA are critical for building neural tissue. In fact, DHA can actually cause the number of neuronal connections to increase.

Prostaglandins are a member of the eicosanoid family. There are "good" eicosanoids and "bad" eicosanoids. Both are necessary for the proper functioning of the inflammatory process in the body. "Good" eicosanoids prevent blood clots, reduce pain, dilate blood vessels, enhance the immune system, and improve brain function. "Bad" eicosanoids promote blood clotting, increase pain, constrict blood vessels, suppress the immune system, and suppress brain function. In general, "good" eicosanoids are anti-inflammatory, and "bad" eicosanoids and pro-inflammatory.

Essential fatty acids play a vital role in how these eicosanoids are produced. Omega-3 fatty acids generally make the "good" eicosanoids, while omega-6 fatty acids lead to the production of "bad" eicosanoids. There are exceptions to this rule, however. LA (omega-6) can lead to the production of "good" eicosanoids through a pathway involving dihomogamma linolenic acid (DGLA). But overall, omega-3s are anti-inflammatory, and omega-6s are pro-inflammatory.

Rudin (1996) states omega-3 fatty acid consumption has decreased 80 percent in the past 100 years while omega-6 fatty acid consumption has increased. Our prehistoric ancestors consumed about a 1:1 omega-6 to omega-3 ratio in their food; however, that ratio in today's diet is more in the range of 10:1 and even as high as 30:1! As you can see, the modern day diet is overloaded in omega-6 fatty acids, and this can lead to the production of "bad" eicosanoids which leads to an increase in inflammation. Trans-fatty acids have also played a role in the deficiency of omega-3 fatty acids, but this problem should no longer exist in the near future thanks to the U.S. government banning the use of these dangerous fats in the American food supply.

A study by B. Deutch done at Aarhus University Denmark and published in the European Journal of Clinical Nutrition in 1995 looked at the level of menstrual pain associated with a low intake of omega-3 fatty acids. The researchers concluded that "results were highly significant and mutually consistent and supported the hypothesis that a higher intake of marine n-3 [omega-3] fatty acids correlates with milder menstrual symptoms (Deutch, 1995, Abstract). Another study by Harel, Biro, Kottenhahn, and Rosenthal (1996) also showed a decrease in menstrual pain with dietary supplementation of omega-3 fatty acids. They conclude "dietary supplementation with omega-3 fatty acids has a beneficial effect on symptoms of dysmenorrhea in adolescents" (Harel et al., 1996, Abstract).

Several studies have shown a decrease in endometriosis symptoms when omega-3 fatty acid consumption is increased. A study done by Covens, Christoper, & Casper (1988) demonstrated this finding in rabbits. The authors showed that "dietary supplementation with fish oil, containing the n-3 polyunsaturated fatty acids EPA and DHA can decrease intraperitoneal PGE2 and PGF2-alpha production and retard endometriotic implant growth in this animal model of endometriosis" (Covens et al., 1988, Abstract). In another study done by Gazvani, Smith, Haggarty, Fowler, and Templeton (2001), the researchers concluded "omega-3 PUFA may have a suppressive effect on the in vitro survival of endometrial cells and omega-3 PUFA may be useful in the management of endometriosis by reducing the inflammatory response and modulating cytokine function" (Abstract). A third study done by Tomio et al. (2013) at the University of Tokyo also showed a protective effect of omega-3 fatty acids in the development of endometriosis. The results of their study showed "that both endogenous and exogenous EPA-derived PUFAs protect against the development of endometriosis through their anti-inflammatory effects and, in particular, the 12/15-LOX-pathway products of EPA may be key mediators to suppress endometriosis" (Abstract).

However, a literature review by Parazzini, Vigano, Candiani, and Fedele (2013) showed omega-3's may not be as effective as originally thought. The authors state, "A protective effect on endometriosis risk has been suggested for vegetable consumption and omega-3 polyunsaturated fatty acid intakes, whereas a negative impact has been reported for red meat consumption and trans fats and coffee intakes, but these findings could not be consistently replicated" (Abstract).

Another study by Missmer, Chavarro, Malspeis, Bertrone-Johnson, and Hornstein (2010) looked at dietary fat consumption and not just the intake of omega-3's. Interestingly, they found that "although total fat consumption was not associated with endometriosis risk, those women in the highest fifth of long-chain omega-3 fatty acid consumption were 22% less likely to be diagnosed with endometriosis compared with those with the lowest fifth of intake…those in the highest quintile of trans-unsaturated fat intake were 48% more likely to be diagnosed with endometriosis…"(Abstract). They concluded that this "provides another disease association that supports efforts to remove trans fat from hydrogenated oils from the food supply" (Abstract).

A study done by Khanaki et al. (2012) performed as a Ph.D. thesis at Tabriz University of Medical Sciences in Iran showed specifically the EPA to AA ratio may be useful in determining the degree of endometriosis present. They conclude "the components and the types of the fatty acids in serum total phospholipids seem not to be a marker for endometriosis, but the EPA/AA ratio is a relevant factor to indicate severity of illness" (Abstract).

The following foods contain excellent sources of omega-3 fatty acids and should be included in the diet of women who suffer from adenomyosis:

    Anchovies
    Canola oil
    Flaxseed
    Herring

Mackerel
Olive oil
Wild salmon
Sardines
Soybean oil
Tuna
Walnuts

Flaxseed – In addition to high levels of omega-3 fatty acids, flaxseed contains the highest known source of lignans in any food. It is one of the best known sources of phytoestrogens and has been shown to inhibit enzymes involved in estrogen production. In addition, studies have shown high levels of estrogen in the urine of those that eat flaxseed on a daily basis (Brooks et al., 2004). In fact, the researchers state "supplementation with flaxseed modifies urinary estrogen metabolite excretion to a greater extent than does supplementation with an equal amount of soy" (Brooks et al., 2004, Abstract). The reason for this is thought to be from the high content of lignans and fiber in flaxseed which help to transport bad estrogen out of the body.

In conclusion, it is clear that omega-3 fatty acids can significantly reduce pain and inflammation. Although omega-6 fatty acids are also necessary for optimum health, today's diet is clearly overloaded with this type of fatty acid and deficient in omega-3. According to Andrew Weil (2000, pg. 88), "if the diet is top-heavy in omega-6 fatty acids, those will compete for a necessary enzyme, blocking the synthesis of DHA." Not only are omega-3 fatty acids vital to reduce inflammation, but there also appears to be a link between a lack of these essential fatty acids and estrogen dominance. For these reasons, women with adenomyosis should definitely include an omega-3 supplement to their daily routine and also increase their consumption of omega-3 rich foods.

Chapter 18 - We Desperately Need More Research!

By now, I'm sure you have come to the conclusion that adenomyosis is a significantly neglected uterine disorder. In a study performed by Taran et al. (2010), the authors concluded that "a better understanding of this disease is required to improve diagnosis and management" (Abstract conclusion section).

One of the main issues is the lack of attention that this disorder has received. Owalbi & Strickler (1977) state "the common association of adenomyosis with more obvious pelvic disease has diminished its significance as a cause of gynaecologic symptoms. Adenomyosis is the addendum to textbook chapters on ectopic endometrium; it is the forgotten process and a neglected diagnosis" (as cited in Taran, 2013, Clinical Phenotype section, para. 2). This is why it is so important to raise awareness of this uterine condition, not only in the medical field, but also in the general public. When I tell people that I had adenomyosis for seventeen years, most of the time they give me a blank stare. But, when I mention endometriosis, they recognize that term. Adenomyosis needs to be as recognizable a term as endometriosis.

One of the biggest problems in researching this disorder has to do with diagnostic criteria. According to Meredith, Sanchez-Ramos, & Kaunitz (2009), it was very difficult to perform a meta-analysis on adenomyosis studies due to the fact that different diagnostic criteria were used. The group states "each study used different definitions of adenomyosis and included studies performed with different ultrasound transducers." (Comments section, para. 5). Accurate information cannot be obtained when the criteria are not consistent. The same group also discussed the actual ultrasound images and the criteria that were used in the meta-analysis saying "most studies included the findings of myometrial heterogeneity or a globular uterus as criteria, while others included the finding of myometrial cysts. Which criterion was most specific for adenomyosis varied between studies" (Comments section, para. 5). With different criteria being used in these studies, we are not able to get an accurate picture of adenomyosis. It is imperative that researchers come up with more stringent criteria in order to get a clearer picture of the disorder.

Another important issue regarding research has to do with the lack of high quality studies. According to Guo (2012), one of the main reasons for lack of reliable knowledge on adenomyosis is the failure of investigators to develop well-controlled studies. Guo states "less than desirable methodological quality of mouse efficacy studies of adenomyosis…could have contributed to the lack of progress in developing novel treatments for adenomyosis" (Methodological Qualities of Published Mouse Efficacy Studies section, para. 2). In addition, Guo (2012) points out that in May, 2012, there were 389 publications of PubMed for adenomyosis as compared to 18,593 for endometriosis. Taran et al. (2013, Abstract, para. 1) states "…despite the clinical importance of adenomyosis, there is little evidence on which to base treatment decisions."

The group concluded in their report that "prospective randomized and controlled studies with larger cohorts, validated and disease-specific symptom questionnaires, noninvasive diagnostic modalities as well as new surgical and interventional alternatives to hysterectomy are required to better understand adenomyosis and to avoid hysterectomy" (Conclusions section, para. 3). No wonder the physicians and ultrasound technologists are unable to diagnose this condition accurately!

During my struggle with adenomyosis, the medications that were prescribed were of very little use to me. I suffered from severe abdominal pain each month, and I was desperate for something to take the edge off the pain. According to Guo (2012), adenomyosis is a "gynecological disorder with a poorly understood pathogenesis" and "more efficacious drugs with better side-effect and cost profiles are sorely needed" (Abstract). Progestins and GnRH are of limited use. According to Guo (2012, Introduction section, para. 2), "progestogenic agents are not very effective, and GnRH agonists...use is restricted by short duration." It has been reported that adenomyosis does not effectively respond to danazol. Clearly, the women who suffer from adenomyosis need more effective ways to manage the pain each month. The current options give minimal relief at best.

Surgical interventions are equally inefficient. Currently, the only way to effectively "cure" adenomyosis is through hysterectomy. Many women opt for this even though they are years away from menopause because they can't take the monthly pain any longer. In addition, many of these women never have children due to the fertility issues involved. This is unacceptable. We need more options for these women.

Another very important reason to determine better treatment options for adenomyosis is the high cost of health care for those who suffer from this disorder. As of 2013, the cost of hysterectomies in the United States were estimated to be 2.1 billion annually (Taran et al., 2013). According to an article published in The Guardian in 2015 by Jessica Glenza, the cost for healthcare the year after a woman is diagnosed with endometriosis was $13,199, and over a ten-year period, the healthcare cost was $26,305 higher than a woman who did not have endometriosis.

Insufficient funding is also a major concern. According to Glenza (2015), endometriosis funding received $7 million in 2014 from the National Institutes of Health (NIH). That number actually went down from 2011 when the funding was double that amount. In addition, Glenza (2015, para. 6) points out that in 2014, "for each person believed to have diabetes in the United States, the NIH spends $35.66 annually. For each woman with endometriosis, the NIH spends $0.92." Those figures are for endometriosis, not adenomyosis! Clearly adenomyosis is a significantly neglected, even ignored, uterine disorder.

Last year, I sent out a petition to the NIH asking for more funding for adenomyosis research. I did receive a very nice and timely response, and they completely understood the frustration that adenomyosis sufferers are dealing with on a daily basis. The explanation for the lack of funding had to do with the lack of applications for well-controlled studies on adenomyosis. After receiving this response, I sent out over fifty petitions to research institutions asking for the development of well-controlled studies on adenomyosis. I asked these researchers to apply for funding through the NIH. As of today, I haven't received a response from any of the petitions. Also, since I am a citizen of the United States, I am appalled at the lack of studies currently being conducted on adenomyosis in this country. As you can see from the list of "Currently Ongoing Studies", the majority are being performed in other countries. I urge research institutions, especially ones in the United States, to develop well-controlled trials and submit their application to the NIH.

Campo et al. (2012) state there is a "renewed interest by the scientific community on an otherwise neglected condition, creating a flurry of research activities leading also to improved knowledge of the relationship between adenomyosis and endometriosis" (Introduction section, para. 7). This is a very encouraging statement, and I hope that this "renewed interest" persists in the coming years. We desperately need more research, better treatment options, and a consensus on the diagnostic criteria for adenomyosis.

Current Ongoing Studies (2016)

Currently recruiting:

What are we Missing? Diagnosing Uterine Adenomyosis Using Ultrasound Elastography
    Location: University of Michigan, Ann Arbor, MI
    For more information, please go to:
    https://clinicaltrials.gov/ct2/show/NCT01992718

The Association Between Adenomyosis/Uterine Myoma and Lower Urinary Tract Symptoms
    Location: Far East Memorial Hospital, Banqiao, Taiwan
    For more information, please go to:
    https://clinicaltrials.gov/ct2/show/NCT02495311

Norwegian Adenomyosis Study I
    Location: Oslo University Hospital, Oslo, Norway
    For more information, please go to:
    https://clinicaltrials.gov/ct2/show/NCT02201719

Norwegian Adenomyosis Study II: Gene Expression Profiling of Adenomyosis
    Location: Oslo University Hospital, Oslo, Norway
    For more information, please go to:
    https://clinicaltrials.gov/ct2/show/NCT02197923

Adenomyosis and Ulipristal Acetate
    Location: AP-HP, Bicêtre Hospital, Le Kremlin Bicêtre, France
    For more information, please go to:
    https://clinicaltrials.gov/ct2/show/NCT02587000

Evaluation of Endometrial Stromal Cell Apoptosis in Adenomyosis
    Location: National Taiwan University Hospital, Taipei, Taiwan
    For more information, please go to:
    https://clinicaltrials.gov/ct2/show/NCT00172588

Efficacy of Trace Elements in the Treatment of Endometriosis: A Pilot Study
    Location: CHU Vésale, Montigny-le-Tilleul, Belgium
    For more information, please go to:
    https://clinicaltrials.gov/ct2/show/NCT02437175

Progestin Treatment for Endometrial Stromal Cells in Adenomyosis
    Location: National Taiwan University Hospital, Taipei, Taiwan
    For more information, please go to:
    https://clinicaltrials.gov/ct2/show/NCT00155051

The Use of Doppler to Diagnose Myometrial Masses
    Location: Cairo University, Cairo, Egypt
    For more information, please go to:
    https://clinicaltrials.gov/ct2/show/NCT01833871

Functional Brain Imaging and Psychological Testing in Women with Chronic Pelvic Pain
    Location: KK Women's and Children's Hospital, Singapore
    For more information, please go to:
    https://clinicaltrials.gov/ct2/show/NCT02160483

Sonohysterography, 3D Ultrasonography and Hysteroscopy in Assessment of Uterine Factor in Cases of Female Infertility
    Location: Cairo University, Cairo, Egypt
    For more information, please go to:
    https://clinicaltrials.gov/ct2/show/NCT02399501

Norwegian Study III – Peristalsis
    Location: Oslo University, Oslo, Norway
    For more information, please go to:
    https://clinicaltrials.gov/ct2/show/NCT02197936

Active but not recruiting:

Vaginal Bromocriptine for Treatment of Adenomyosis
    Location: Mayo Clinic, Rochester, MN
    For more information, please go to:
    https://clinicaltrials.gov/ct2/show/NCT01821001

LNG-IUS for Treatment of Dysmenorrhea
    Location: Egypt
    For more information, please go to:
    https://clinicaltrials.gov/ct2/show/NCT01601366

Proliferation of Endometrial Stromal Cells in Adenomyosis
    Location: National Taiwan University Hospital, Taipei, Taiwan
    For more information, please go to:
    https://clinicaltrials.gov/ct2/show/NCT00173212

The Impact of Gynecological Surgery on Ovarian Function in Women of Reproductive Age: Postoperative Changes of Serum Anti-Müllerian Hormone (AMH)
    Location: Samsung Medical Center, South Korea
    For more information, please go to:
    https://clinicaltrials.gov/ct2/show/NCT00928044

Recently Completed:

The Diagnostic Accuracy of Hysteroscopic Endomyometrial Biopsy in Adenomyosis
    Location: Woman's Health University Hospital, Cairo, Egypt
    For more information, please go to:
    https://clinicaltrials.gov/ct2/show/NCT02340533

Aromatase Inhibitors or GnRH-a for Uterine Adenomyosis
    Location: Mansoura University Hospital, Mansoura, Egypt
    For more information, please go to:
    https://clinicaltrials.gov/ct2/show/NCT01218581

AMH (Anti-Müllerian Hormone) Level Change During Treatment with GnRH Agonist
    Location: University Magna Graecia, Catanzaro, Italy
    For more information, please go to:
    https://clinicaltrials.gov/ct2/show/NCT02086279

Tactile Electrosurgical Ablation in Cases of Dysfunctional Uterine Bleeding
    Location: Woman's Health Hospital, Assiut University, Assiut, Egypt
    For more information, please go to:
    https://clinicaltrials.gov/ct2/show/NCT02248194

Use of Dexamethasone in Uterine Artery Embolization
    Location: Severance Hospital, Seoul, Korea
    For more information, please go to:
    https://clinicaltrials.gov/ct2/show/NCT02056717

Uterine Artery Embolization for Symptomatic Fibroids
    Location: University of Manitoba, Winnipeg, Manitoba, Canada
    For more information, please go to:
    https://clinicaltrials.gov/ct2/show/NCT00354471

Efficacy of Acupuncture on Chronic Pelvic Pain in Women with Endometriosis or Adenomyosis
    Location: East West Neo Medical Center, Seoul, Korea
    For more information, please go to:
    https://clinicaltrials.gov/ct2/show/NCT01259180

Status Unknown:

Health-Related QoL Among Women Receiving Hysterectomy in National Taiwan University Hospital
    Location: National Taiwan University Hospital, Taipei, Taiwan
    For more information, please go to:
    https://clinicaltrials.gov/ct2/show/NCT00155870

Abbreviations

4-MBC – 4-methylbenzylidine camphor
β-HCH – β-hexachlorocyclohexane
AA – Arachidonic acid
ATP – Adenosine tri-phosphate
BCP – Birth control pill
BHA – Butylated hydroxyanisole
BPA – Bisphenol A
CA19-9 – Cancer antigen 19-9
CA125 – Cancer antigen 125
CAPE – Caffeic acid phenethyl ester
COX2 – Cyclo-oxygenase
D&C – Dilation and curettage
DDT – Dichlorodiphenyltrichloroethane
DEHP – di(2-ethylhexyl) phthalate
DES – Diethylstilbestrol
DGLA – Dihomogamma linolenic acid
DHA – Docosahexanoic acid
DIM - Diindolylmethane
E1 - Estrone
E2 - Estradiol
E3 - Estriol
EFA – Essential fatty acid or Endometriosis Foundation of America
EMI – Endometrial myometrial interface
EPA – Eicosapentenoic acid or Environmental Protection Agency
ERα – Estrogen receptor alpha
ERβ – Estrogen receptor beta
FSH – Follicle-stimulating hormone
GLA – Gamma linoleic acid
GnRH – Gonadotropin-releasing hormone
hCG – Human chorionic gonadotropin
HRT – Hormone replacement therapy
I3C - Indole-3-carbinol
IBS – Irritable bowel syndrome
IL-6 – Interleukin-6
IUD – Intrauterine device
IV - Intravenous
IVF – In vitro fertilization
JZ – Junctional zone
LA – Linoleic acid

LH – Luteinizing hormone
LNA – Alpha-linolenic acid
MAOI – Monoamine oxidase inhibitor
MMP2 – Matrix metalloproteinase
MRgFUS – Magnetic resonance-guided focused ultrasound
MRI – Magnetic resonance imaging
MRSA – Methicillin-resistant staphylococcus aureus
NAC – N-acetyl cysteine
NSAID – Non-steroidal anti-inflammatory drug
OCP – Organochlorine pesticide
PBB – Polybrominated biphenyl
PCB – Polychlorinated biphenyl
PCOS – Polycystic ovarian syndrome
PGE2 – Prostaglandin E2
PGF2 – Prostaglandin F2 alpha
PID – Pelvic inflammatory disease
PMDD – Premenstrual dysphoric disorder
PUFA – Polyunsaturated fatty acid
RCT – Randomized controlled trial
SAMe – S-adenosyl methionine
TVS – Transvaginal sonogram
UAE – Uterine artery embolization
US – Ultrasound
VEGF – Vascular endothelial growth factor

Definitions

β-hexachlorocyclohexane (β-HCH) – a type of organochlorine pesticide.

Adenocarcinoma – cancer that arises from glandular tissue.

Adenomyoma – abnormal mass of endometrial tissue found within the myometrium. An adenomyoma is usually benign and is associated with adenomyosis.

Adenosine tri-phosphate (ATP) – a substance that is a part of energy transportation in cells as a part of the process of metabolism.

Adhesion – abnormal union of two separate tissues as a result of inflammation.

Adrenal fatigue – condition where the adrenals are not functioning at the optimum level. It is characterized by unrefreshing sleep and is usually caused my chronic stress or chronic infection.

Agonist – a chemical that stimulates action.

Alpha-linolenic acid (LNA) – a type of omega-3 fatty acid that can be converted to EPA and DHA in the body. It is an essential fatty acid (must be included in the diet).

Amenorrhea – absence of menstruation.

Anemia – low levels of hemoglobin present in red blood cells. Since hemoglobin is involved in the transport of oxygen throughout the body, low levels can cause fatigue, dizziness, headache, shortness of breath, and cold intolerance. One cause of anemia is excessive blood loss from menstruation.

Angiogenesis – the growth of new blood vessels in the human body.

Anovulation – failure to release an egg from the ovary.

Antagonist – a substance that interferes with the action of another substance.

Antibacterial – substance that kills bacteria.

Antifungal – substance that kills fungi.

Antioxidant – a molecule that inhibits oxidation, thereby reducing free radical formation.

Aphrodisiac – substance that increases sexual desire.

Apoptosis – programmed cell death necessary for the proper functioning of the human body.

Arachidonic acid (AA) – a type of omega-6 fatty acid that is heavily involved in the inflammatory process. This fatty acid is also a vasodilator.

Aromatase – enzyme that converts androgens to estrogen in the body.

Astringent – a substance that shrinks body tissues.

Bioactivity – the effect of a substance on living tissue.

Bioidentical progesterone cream – progesterone that is identical to endogenous progesterone on a molecular level.

Biopsy – removal of a small piece of tissue from the body. It is then viewed under a microscope to rule out an abnormality.

Cancer antigen 19-9 (CA19-9) – tumor marker for pancreatic cancer.

Cancer antigen 125 (CA125) – the CA125 test is used to look for early signs of ovarian cancer.

Carcinogen – substance that causes cancer.

Carminative – a substance that expels gas.

Cervix – cylindrical shaped tissue that separates the uterus from the vagina.

Chelator – a compound that can bind to a metal. Chelators are used to help eliminate metal toxins from the body.

Circadian rhythm – a 24-hour cycle of physical and mental changes that respond to light and dark.

Cirrhosis – damage to the liver that causes it to function suboptimally.

Cohort – a group of people.

Corpus luteum – formed from an ovarian follicle after the egg has been released. It secretes progesterone in order to support a pregnancy; however, if the egg is not fertilized, the corpus luteum will degenerate.

Cystic – related to or containing cysts.

Cytochrome P450 – these hemoproteins are involved in the metabolism of toxins in the body. Most of these hemoproteins are found in the liver.

Detoxification cleanse – process of using nutrients to help eliminate toxins from the body.

Dienogest – semi-synthetic progestogen. It has been used to treat endometriosis under the name "Visanne".

Diuretic – substance that encourages fluid loss from the body and increases urine output.

Diverticulitis – infected or inflamed pouches (diverticula) on the wall of the colon. Symptoms include gas, bloating, constipation, diarrhea, abdominal pain, loss of appetite, and nausea.

Docosahexanoic acid (DHA) – a type of omega-3 fatty acid that is found in cold water fatty fish.

Dysmenorrhea – painful menstrual bleeding.

Echotexture – characteristic pattern seen on radiology images.

Ectopic – occurring in an abnormal place; out of position.

Ectopic pregnancy – pregnancy that occurs outside of the uterus, usually in the fallopian tube. This is a dangerous condition and should be promptly treated as it can cause internal bleeding and possible death.

Eicosanoid – molecule that is made from omega-3 and omega-6 fatty acids. Prostaglandins, leukotrienes, thromboxanes, and lipoxins are all eicosanoids. They are heavily involved in the inflammatory process in the body.

Eicosapentenoic acid (EPA) – a type of omega-3 fatty acid that is found in cold water fatty fish.

Endocrine disruptor – chemicals that cause hormonal imbalance by interfering with the endocrine system.

Endogenous – caused by internal factors; having an internal cause. Endogenous progesterone is progesterone manufactured by the human body.

Endometrial carcinoma – uterine cancer that begins in the endometrium.

Endometrioma – cyst is formed in the ovaries by displaced endometrial tissue that is seen in endometriosis patients. Also called a "chocolate cyst" because of its deep red/brown appearance.

Epithelium – closely packed cells that line the interior and exterior surfaces of the body. An example is the skin. It is one of the four major tissue types of the human body.

Essential fatty acid (EFA) – fats that can't be synthesized in the human body and must be included in the diet. LNA and LA are essential fatty acids.

Estradiol (E2) – the most potent form of estrogen. It is the predominant form of estrogen in a woman's body during the reproductive years. The level of estradiol drops after menopause.

Estriol (E3) – a type of estrogen that is produced by the placenta and is abundant during pregnancy.

Estrone (E1) – least abundant type of estrogen. It is less potent than estradiol and is the major form of estrogen found in menopausal women. Estrone can be converted into estradiol.

Expectorant – a substance that enhances the expulsion of mucus.

Fallopian tube – tube connecting the ovary to the uterus. The egg travels down this tube after being released from the ovarian follicle.

Fibrocystic disease (breast) – non-cancerous cysts in the breast. Can be solid (fibrosis) or fluid-filled.

Fibroid – benign tumor of uterine smooth muscle. Also referred to as a leiomyoma, it can cause heavy periods, infertility, and anemia.

Follicle-stimulating hormone (FSH) – hormone produced in the anterior pituitary gland. FSH is responsible for the maturation of the follicle in the ovary.

Free radical – an atom with at least one unpaired electron. It is highly reactive and can damage cells.

Gamma linoleic acid (GLA) – a type of omega-6 fatty acid. GLA can be converted into AA in the body. A good source of this fatty acid is evening primrose oil.

Gonadotropin – a hormone that stimulates the gonads. FSH and LH are examples.

Hepatitis – inflammation of the liver.

Hepatobiliary – refers to the combination of the liver, gallbladder, and bile ducts.

Herbicide – chemical used to kill unwanted plants.

HOX genes – genes that control the development of the basic structure of the body. Also called homeotic genes.

Hyperperistalsis (uterus) – condition where uterine contractions are more frequent than those seen in a normal uterus.

Hyperplastic – increase in the number of normal cells in an organ or tissue. Cells may also be larger than normal.

Hyperprolactinemia – higher than normal levels of prolactin in a female's body. Can cause oligomenorrhea, amenorrhea, and infertility.

Hypertrophic – excessive growth of an organ or tissue.

Hypothyroidism – an underactive thyroid. The gland doesn't produce enough thyroid hormone which causes fatigue, weight gain, depression, and constipation.

Implantation – in the uterus, this refers to the adherence of a fertilized egg to the wall of the uterus.

In vitro – tests conducted in an artificial environment outside of a living organism. Latin for "within the glass".

In vivo – tests performed on living tissue. Latin for "within the living".

Insecticide - chemical used to kill insects.

Interleukin 6 (IL-6) - chemicals are actively involved in the inflammatory process and act as pyrogens (induce fevers).

Irritable bowel syndrome (IBS) - disorder of the colon that can cause abdominal pain, cramping, bloating, constipation and/or diarrhea. IBS is a diagnosis of exclusion which means that the physician must rule out all other known causes of these symptoms before this diagnosis can be given. IBS is a functional disorder of the colon due to abnormal peristalsis, and it is not life-threatening.

Isoflavones – strong antioxidants that have estrogen-like activity in the body.

Laxative – a substance that loosens stools and promotes bowel movements.

Leiomyoma – see "Fibroid".

Lignans – substances found in plants. Bacteria break down lignans in the intestinal tract to substances that have weak estrogen activity. Lignans are the main source of phytoestrogens in the diet.

Linoleic acid (LA) – a type of omega-6 fatty acid that can be converted to GLA and then to AA in the body. This type of fatty acid is essential (must be included in the diet).

Luteal insufficiency – condition where the uterine lining fails to grow properly each month. This is due to low progesterone levels or the failure of the uterine lining to respond properly to progesterone. This condition may cause fertility issues and is also referred to as "luteal phase defect".

Luteinizing hormone (LH) – hormone produced in the anterior pituitary gland. A surge in LH occurs in the last half of the menstrual cycle and is responsible for ovulation and the development of the corpus luteum.

Macrophage – a type of white blood cell that is large and is involved in the destruction of foreign invaders, such as bacteria, in the body.

Menarche – the first menstrual cycle.

Menorrhagia – abnormally heavy menstrual bleeding.

Meta-analysis – an analysis that uses statistics to combine findings from two or more studies.

Metabolite – an intermediate substance produced during metabolism.

Microcyst – a cyst that can only be seen with a microscope.

Monoamine oxidase inhibitor (MAOI) – a type of antidepressant.

Mucilage – a viscous or gelatin-like substance.

Mucilaginous – a sticky substance that secretes mucilage.

Müllerian ducts – embryonic ducts that develop into fallopian tubes, uterus, cervix, and vagina.

Mutation – a permanent change in a DNA sequence.

Myometrial ectopic pregnancy – pregnancy that occurs within the uterine wall. This condition is rare, but it can cause uterine rupture.

Neoplastic – abnormal growth of tissue that can be either malignant or benign.

Oligomenorrhea – infrequent or very light menstrual periods.

Ovarian cyst – solid or fluid-filled sac on the surface or within an ovary. Most do not cause symptoms; however, if the cysts are large or have ruptured, they can cause pelvic pain, painful intercourse, nausea, and vomiting.

Ovarian follicles – a spherical group of cells found in the ovary. They secrete hormones and hold oocytes which eventually develop into eggs.

Oxytocin – hormone that helps to regulate childbirth and breast-feeding. It is produced in the hypothalamus and stored in the posterior pituitary gland.

Pathogenesis – the mechanism of the development of a disease.

Pelvic inflammatory disease (PID) - infection is caused by bacteria that has made its way through the cervix and into the rest of the female reproductive tract. Symptoms include lower abdominal pain, abnormal vaginal discharge, nausea, and vomiting. It is usually sexually transmitted.

Peristalsis – involuntary rhythmic contractions that move contents through a tubular organ.

Peritoneum – the membrane that lines the walls of the abdomen and protects the abdominal organs.

Pesticide – chemical that kills any kind of pest. Herbicides and insecticides are two types of pesticides.

Pituitary gland – pea-sized gland located at the base of the brain. It controls the functioning of other endocrine glands and is involved in the production of several different hormones in the human body. Also referred to as the "master gland".

Polycystic ovarian syndrome (PCOS) – a condition where many small cysts develop on the ovaries. This is due to a hormonal imbalance caused by excessive levels of androgens. Symptoms include excess body hair, weight gain, infertility, and irregular periods.

Polyunsaturated fatty acid (PUFA) – type of fat that has more than one unsaturated carbon bond. Examples are omega-3 and omega-6 fatty acids. These fats are liquid at room temperature and solid when refrigerated.

Pre-menstrual dysphoric disorder (PMDD) – a severe form of premenstrual syndrome (PMS).

Proanthocyanidins – a type of flavonoid found in plants. They are antioxidants and are known to be beneficial in cardiovascular disease, diabetes, and cancer.

Progestins – synthetic progestogens.

Progestogens – steroid hormones that bind to the progesterone receptors and activate them. Progesterone is the most well-known progestogen.

Prolactin – hormone that stimulates the production of breast milk. It is made by the pituitary gland.

Prospective trials – study that follows a group over a set period of time.

Prostaglandin – a type of lipid that controls the contraction and relaxation of smooth muscle, modulates inflammation, and regulates blood flow. It is made from arachidonic acid, a type of omega-6 fatty acid.

Randomized controlled trials – studies where people are randomly placed in groups that receive different treatments. An example is a study of the usefulness/side effects of a medication. One group is a control group that will receive a placebo, and the other group is the experimental group that will receive the medication. Those involved in the study do not know who is receiving the placebo and who is receiving the actual medication. This is the most common type of scientific study performed since it minimizes bias.

Sedative – a substance that induces sleep.

Speculum – an instrument that looks like the "beak of a duck" and is used to spread open the walls of the vagina.

Submucosal – connective tissue that lies beneath a mucous membrane.

Subperitoneal – located beneath the peritoneum.

Surfactant – a substance that reduces the surface tension of a liquid allowing it to foam and penetrate solids.

T-cells – a type of white blood cell that is heavily involved in immune system function.

Tamoxifen – a medicine used in the treatment of breast cancer.

Tonic – a substance that promotes general health.

Trans-fatty acid – manufactured fatty acids that are dangerous to health. These fats are created through a process called hydrogenation.

Uterine polyp – mass that originates from the endometrium. It can be flat up against the uterine wall or may be pedunculated (on a stalk). Polyps can grow up to several centimeters and may be associated with heavy menstrual bleeding. Also referred to as an "endometrial polyp".

Vascularization – development of blood vessels through natural or surgical means.

References

Adb-Allah, A. R. A., El-Sayed, E. S. M., Abdel-Wahab, M. H., & Hamada, F. M. A. (2003). Effect of melatonin on estrogen and progesterone receptors in relation to uterine contraction in rats. *Pharmacological Research, 47(4),* 349-54. doi: 10.1016/S1043-6618(03)00014-8

Bacciottini, L., Falchetti, A., Pampaloni, B, Bartolini, E., Carossino, A. M., & Brandi, M. L. (2007). Phytoestrogens: Food or drug? *Clinical Cases in Mineral and Bone Metabolism, 4(2),* 123-130. Retrieved from http://www.ncbi.nlm.gov/pmc/articles/PMC2781234

Barrett, J. R. (2006). The science of soy: What do we really know? *Environmental Health Perspectives, 114(6),* A352-A358. Retrieved from. http://www.ncbi.nlm.nih.gov/pmc/articles/PMC1480510/

Barton-Schuster, D. (2015) Herbs and supplements with estrogen action Q&A. Message posted to http://natural-fertility-info/herbs-and-with-supplements estrogen-action-qa.html

Bazot, M., Cortez, A., Darai, E., Rouger, J., Chopier, J., Antoine, J. M., & Uzan, S. (2001). Ultrasonography compared with magnetic resonance imaging for the diagnosis of adenomyosis: correlation with histopathology. *Human Reproduction, 16(11),* 2427-33. Retrieved from http://www.ncbi.nlm.nih.gov/pubmed/11679533

Beck, V., Unterrieder, E., Krenn, L., Kubelka, W., & Jungbauer, A. (2003). Comparison of hormonal activity (estrogen, androgen and progestin) of standardized plant extracts for large scale use in hormone replacement therapy. *Journal of Steroid Biochemistry and Molecular Biology, 84(2-3),* 259-68. Retrieved from http://www.ncbi.nlm.nih.gov/pubmed/12711012

Behera, M. A., & Gest, T. R. (2011). Uterus anatomy. In *Medscape.* Retrieved from http://emedicine.medscape.com/article/1949215-overview#a1

Benagiano, G. P., Brosens, I. A., Carrara, S., & Filippi, V. (2010). Adenomyosis. In *The Global Library of Women's Medicine, ISSN:1756-2228.* doi: 10.3843/GLOWM.10460

Benagiano, G., Brosens, I., & Carrara, S. (2009). Adenomyosis: New knowledge is generating new treatment strategies. *Women's Health, 5(3),* 297-311. Retrieved from http://www.medscape.com/viewarticle/703820_5

Bergner, P. (2001). Glycyrrhiza: Licorice root and testosterone. *Medical Herbalism, 11(3),* 11-12. Retrieved from http://www.medherb.com/Materia_Medica/Glycyrrhiza_-_Licorice_root_and_testosterone.htm

Beta-catenin. Retrieved April 13, 2015 from Wikipedia: http://en.wikipedia.org/wiki/Beta-catenin

Bioscience Technology (2013). Closing in on cause of adenomyosis Retrieved from http://www.biosciencetechnology.com/news/2013/10/closing-cause-adenomyosis

Boue, S. M., Wiese, T. E., Nehls, S., Burow, M. E., Elliott, S., Carter-Wientjes, C. H.,...Cleveland, T. E. (2003). Evaluation of the estrogenic effects of legume extracts containing phytoestrogens. *Journal of Agricultural and Food Chemistry, 51(8),* 2193-9. Retrieved from http://www.ncbi.nlm.nih.gov/pubmed/12670155

Bratby, M. J., & Walker, M. J. (2009). Uterine artery embolization for symptomatic adenomyosis – mid-term results. *European Journal of Radiology, 70(1),* 128-132. doi: http://dx.doi.org/10.1016/j.ejrad.2007.12.009

Bromley, B., Shipp, T. D., & Benacerraf, B. (2000). Adenomyosis: Sonographic findings and diagnostic accuracy. *Journal of Ultrasound in Medicine, 19,* 529-534. Retrieved from http://www.jultrasoundmed.org/content/19/8/529.full.pdf

Brooks, J. D., Ward, W. E., Lewis, J. E., Hilditch, J., Nickell, L., Wong, E., & Thompson, L. U. (2004). Supplementation with flaxseed alters estrogen metabolism in postmenopausal women to a greater extent than does supplementation with an equal amount of soy. *American Journal of Clinical Nutrition, 79(2),* 318-325. Retrieved from http://ajcn.nutrition.org/content/79/2/318.full

Bulayeva, N., & Watson, C. (2004). Xenoestrogen-induced ERK-1 and ERK-2 activation via multiple membrane-initiated signaling pathways. *Environmental Health Perspectives, 112(15),* 1481-87. Retrieved from http://www.bvsde.paho.org/bvsacd/ehp/v112-15/p1481.pdf

Campo, S., Campo, V., & Benagiano, G. (2012). Infertility and adenomyosis. *Obstetrics and Gynecology International, Volume 2012, article ID 786132.* doi: 10.1155/2012/786132

Cho, S., Nam, A., Kim, H., Chay, D., Park, K., Cho, D.J.,...Lee, B. (2008). Clinical Effects of the levonorgestrel-releasing intrauterine device in patients with adenomyosis. *American Journal of Obstetrics and Gynecology, 198(4),* 373, e1-7. doi: 10.1016/j.ajog.2007.10.798

Cleveland Clinic (2016). Rosemary Supplement Review. Retrieved from http://www.clevelandclinicwellness.com/Features/Pages/rosemary.aspx

Covens, A. L., Christoper, P., & Casper, R. F. (1988). The effect of dietary supplementation with fish oil fatty acids on surgically induced endometriosis in the rabbit. *Fertility and Sterility (Impact Factor 4.17), 49(4),* 698-703. Retrieved from http://www.researchgate.net/publication/20324462_The_effect_of_dietary_supplementation_with_f ish_oil_fatty_acids_on_surgically_induced_endometriosis_in_the_ rabbit

Davis, S. R., Dalais, F. S., Simpson, E. R., & Murkies, A. L. (1999). Phytoestrogens in health and disease. *Recent Progress in Hormone Research, 54,* 185-210, discussion 210-1. Retrieved from http://www.ncbi.nlm.nih.gov/pubmed/10548876

de Souza, N. M., Brosens, J. J., Schwieso, J. E., Paraschos, T., & Winston, R. M. (1995). The potential value of magnetic resonance imaging in infertility. *Clinical Radiology, 50(2),* 75-9. Retrieved from http://www.ncbi.nlm.nih.gov/pubmed/7867272

Deutch, B. (1995). Menstrual pain in Danish women correlated with low n-3 polyunsaturated fatty acid intake. *European Journal of Clinical Nutrition, 49(7),* 508-16. Retrieved from http://www.researchgate.net/publication/15609638_Menstrual_pain_in_Danish_women_correlated _with_low_n-3_polyunsaturated_fatty_acid_intake

Dueholm, M., Lundorf, E., Hansen, E.S., Sorensen, J. S., Ledertoug, S., & Olesen, F. (2001). Magnetic resonance imaging and transvaginal ultrasonography for the diagnosis of adenomyosis. *Fertility and Sterility, 76,* 588-594.doi: http://dx.doi.org/10.1016/Soo15-0282(01)01962-8

Endometriosis Foundation of America. (2015). Endometriosis. Retrieved from http://www.endofound.org/endometriosis

Estrogen Dominance. Retrieved April 13, 2015 from Wikipedia: http://en.wikipedia.org/wiki/Estrogen_dominance

Eubanks, M. (2004). The safety of xenoestrogens. *Environmental Health Perspectives, 112(15),* A897. Retrieved from http://www.ncbi.nlm.gov/pmc/articles/PMC1247635

Exacoustos, C., Brienza, L., DiGiovanni, A., Szabolcs, B., Romanini, M. E., Zupi, E., & Arduini, D. (2011). Adenomyosis: Three dimensional sonographic findings of the junctional zone and correlation with histology. *Ultrasound in Obstetrics and Gynecology, 37(4),* 471-9. doi: 10.1002/uog.8900

Fedele, L., Bianchi, S., Zonotti, F., Marchini, M., & Candiani, G. B. (1993). Fertility after conservative surgery for adenomyomas. *Human Reproduction, 8(10),* 1708-1710. Retrieved from http://www.ncbi.nlm.nih.gov/pubmed/8300834

Focused Ultrasound Foundation. (2015). Adenomyosis. Retrieved from http://www.fusfoundation.org/diseases-and-conditions/women-s-health/adenomyosis

Frezza, M., Tritapepe, R., Pozzato, G., & De Padova, C. (1998). Prevention of s-adenosylmethionine of estrogen-induced hepatobiliary toxicity in susceptible women. *American Journal of Gastroenterology, 83(10),* 1098-102. Retrieved from http://www.ncbi.nlm.nih.gov/pubmed/3421220

Fry, M. (1995). Reproductive effects in birds exposed to pesticides and industrial chemicals. *Environmental Health Perspectives, 103(Suppl 7),* 165-171. Retrieved from http://www.ncbi.nlm.nih.gov/PMC/articles/PMC1518881/pdf/envhper00367-0160.pdf

Fukunishi, H., Funaki, K., Sawada, K., Yamaguchi, K., Tetsuo, M., & Yasushi, K. (2008). Early results of magnetic resonance-guided focused ultrasound surgery of adenomyosis: analysis of 20 cases. *Journal of Minimally Invasive Gynecology, 15(5),* 571-579. doi: 10.1016/j.jmig.2008.06.010

Furuhashi, M., Miyabe, Y., Katsumata, Y., Oda, H., & Imai, N. (1998). Comparison of complications of vaginal hysterectomy in patients with leiomyomas and in patients with adenomyosis. *Archives of Gynecology and Obstetrics, 262(1-2),* 69-73. Retrieved from http://ncbi.nlm.nih.gov/pubmed/9836003

Gazvani, M. R., Smith, L., Haggarty, P., Fowler, P.A., & Templeton, A. (2001). High omega-3:omega-6 fatty acid ratios in culture medium reduce endometrial-cell survival in combined endometrial gland and stromal cell cultures from women with and without endometriosis. *Fertility and Sterility, 76(4),* 717-22. Retrieved from http://www.ncbi.nlm.nih.gov/pubmed/11591404

Glenza, J. (2015). Endometriosis often ignored as millions of American women suffer. *The Guardian.* Retrieved from http://www.the guardian.com/us-news/2015/sep/27/endometriosis-ignored-federal-research-funding

Gordts, S., Brosens, J. J., Fusi, L., Benagiano, G., & Brosens, I. (2008). Uterine adenomyosis: A need for uniform terminology and consensus classification. *Reproductive BioMedicine Online, 17(2),* 244-8. Retrieved from http://www.ncbi.nlm.nih.gov/pubmed/18681999

Guo, S. W. (2012). Methodological issues in preclinical mouse efficacy studies of adenomyosis. *Current Obstetrics and Gynecology Reports, 1,* 138-145. doi: 10.1007/s13669-012-0018-3

Harel, Z., Biro, F. M., Kottenhahn, R. K., & Rosenthal, S. L. (1996). Supplementation with omega-3 polyunsaturated fatty acids in the management of dysmenorrhea in adolescents. *American Journal of Obstetrics and Gynecology, 174(4),* 1335-8. doi: 10.1016/S0002-9378(96)70681-6

Hayes, T., Haston, K., Tsui, M., Hoang, A., Haeffele, C., & Vonk, A. (2003). Atrazine-induced hermaphroditism at 0.1 ppb in American leopard frogs (Ranna pipiens): laboratory and field evidence. *Environmental Health Perspectives, 111(4),* 568-575. Retrieved from http://www.ncbi.nlm.nih.gov/pubmed/PMC1241446

Hirata, T., Izumi, G., Takamura, M., Saito, A., Nakazawa, A., Harada, M.,… Osuga, Y. (2014) Efficacy of dienogest in the treatment of symptomatic adenomyosis: A pilot study. *Gynecology and Endocrinology,* 1-4. Retrieved from http://www.ncbi.nlm.nih.gov/pubmed/24905725

Hiroyuki, M., Ideda, T., Kajita, K., Fujioka, K., Mori, I., Okada, H.,… Ishizuka, T. (2012). Effect of royal jelly ingestion for six months on healthy volunteers. *Nutrition Journal, 11,* 77. doi: 10.1186/1475-2891-11-77

Huang, W. H., Yang, T. S., & Yuan, C. C. (1998). Successful pregnancy after treatment of deep adenomyosis with cytoreductive surgery and subsequent gonadotropin-releasing hormone agonist: A case report. *Zhonghua Yi Xue Za Zhi, 61(12),* 726-9. Retrieved from http://www.ncbi.nlm.nih.gov/pubmed/9884446

Humphrey, C. D. (1998). Phytoestrogens and human health effects: Weighing up the current evidence. *Natural Toxins, 6(2),* 51-9. Retrieved from http://www.ncbi.nlm.nih.gov/pubmed/9888630

Jackson-Michel, S. (2015). Herbs for estrogen dominance. Retrieved from http://www.livestrong.com/article/123225-herbs-estrogen-dominance/

Jefferson, W. N., Padilla-Banks, E., & Newbold, R. R. (2007). Disruption of The developing female reproductive system by phytoestrogens: Genistein as an example. *Molecular Nutrition and Food Research, 51(7),* 832-844. doi: 10.1002/mnfr.200600258

Johnston, I. M., & Johnston, J. R. (1990). Flaxseed (Linseed) oil and the power of omega-3. Los Angeles: Keats Publishing.

Jung, B. I., Kim, M. S., Kim, H. A., Kim, D., Yang, J., Her, S., & Song, Y.S. (2010). Caffeic acid phenethylester, a component of beehive propolis, is a novel selective estrogen receptor modulator. *Phytotherapy Research, 24(2),* 295-300. doi: 10.1002/ptr.2966

Kaye, J. (2011). Xenoestrogens. Retrieved from http://www.drjosephkaye.com/2011/10/14/xenoestrogens/

Khanaki, K., Nouri, M., Ardekani, A. M., Ghassemzadeh, A., Shahnazi, V., Sadeqhi, M. R.,...Rahimipour, A. (2012). Evaluation of the relationship between endometriosis and omega-3 and omega-6 polyunsaturated fatty acids. *Iranian Biomedical Journal, 16(1),* 38-43. doi: 10.6091/IBJ.1025.2012

Kijma, I., Phung, S., Hur, G., Kwok, S. L., & Chen, S. (2006). Grape seed extract is an aromatase inhibitor and a suppressor of aromatase expression. *Cancer Research, 66(11),* 5960-7. Retrieved from http://www.ncbi.nlm.nih.gov/pubmed/16740737

Kim, K.A., Yoon, S. W., Lee, C., Seong, S. J., Yoon, B. S., & Park, H. (2011). Short-term results of magnetic resonance imaging-guided focused ultrasound surgery for patients with adenomyosis: Symptomatic relief and pain reduction. *Fertility and Sterility, 95(3),* 1152-1155. doi: 10.1016/j.fertnstert.2010.09.024

Kim, M. J., Park, J. H., Kwon, D. Y., Yang, H. J., Kim da, S., Kang, S.,... Park, S. (2014). The supplementation of Korean mistletoe water extracts reduces hot flushes, dyslipidemia, hepatic steatosis, and muscle loss in ovariectomized rats. *Experimental Biology and Medicine, 240(4),* 477-87. doi: 10.1177/1535370214551693

Kunz, G., Herbertz, M., Beil, D., Huppert, P., & Leyendecker, G. (2007). Adenomyosis as a disorder of the early and late human reproductive period. *Reproductive Biomedicine Online, 15(6),* 681-5. Retrieved from http://ncbi.nlm.nih.gov/pubmed/18062865

Kurzer, M. S. (2002). Hormonal effects of soy in premenopausal women and men. *Journal of Nutrition, 132(3),* 570S-573S. Retrieved from http://www.ncbi.nlm.nih.gov/pubmed/11880595

Lam, M. (2015a). Estrogen dominance – Part 1. Retrieved from http://www.drlam/com/Articles/Estrogen_Dominance.asp

Lam, M. (2015b). Estrogen dominance – Part 2. Retrieved from http://www.drlam.com/blog/estrogen-dominance-part-2/1781/

Lam, M. (2015c). How and when did estrogen dominance arise? Retrieved from http://www.biomediclabs.com/health-articles/

LaRue, A. (2012). Xenoestrogens – What are they? How to avoid them. *Women in Balance Institute: National College of Natural Medicine.* Retrieved from http://womeninbalance.org/2012/10/26/xenoestrogens-what-are-they-how-to-avoid-them/

Lee, J. R. (2016). Four simple steps for balancing hormones naturally. Retrieved from http://www.johnleemd.com

Leyendecker, G., Kunz, G., Wildt, L., Beil, D., & Deininger, H. (1996). Uterine hyperperistalsis and dysperistalsis as dysfunctions of the mechanism of rapid sperm transport in patients with endometriosis and infertility. *Human Reproduction, 11(7),* 1542-51. Retrieved from http://www.ncbi.nlm.nih.gov/pubmed/8671502

Lin, J., Sun, C., & Li, R. (1999). Gonadotropin releasing hormone agonists in the treatment of adenomyosis with infertility. *Zhonghua Fu Chan Ke Za Zhi, 34(4),* 214-16. Retrieved from http://www.ncbi.nlm.nih.gov/pubmed/11326917

Liske, E., Hanggi, M. D., & Henneicke-von Zepelin, H. H., (2002). Physiological investigation of a unique extract of black cohosh (cimicifugae racemosae rhizoma): A 6-month clinical study demonstrates no systemic estrogenic effect. *Journal of Women's Health & Gender-Based Medicine, 11,* 163-174. Retrieved from http://www.ncbi.nlm.nih.gov/pubmed/11975864

Liu, J., Burdette, J. E., & Xu, H. (2001). Evaluation of estrogenic activity of plant extracts for the potential treatment of menopausal symptoms. *Journal of Agricultural and Food Chemistry, 49,* 2472-2479. Retrieved from http://www.ncbi.nlm.nih.gov/pubmed/11368622

Liu, J. J., Duan, H., & Wang, S. (2013). Expression of nitric oxide in uterine junctional zone of patients with adenomyosis. *Zhonghua Fu Chan Ke Za Zhi, 48(7),* 504-7. Retrieved from http://www.ncbi.nlm.nih.gov/pubmed/24284220

Loffer, F. D. (1995). Endometrial ablation and resection. *Current Opinion in Obstetrics and Gynecology, 7(4),* 290-4. Retrieved from http://www.ncbi.nlm.nih.gov/pubmed/7578969

Mansukhani, N., Unni, J., Dua, M., Darbari, R., Malik, S., Verma, S., & Bathla, S. (2013). Are women satisfied when using levonorgestrel-releasing uterine system for treatment of abnormal uterine bleeding? *Journal of Mid-Life Health, 4(1),* 31-35. doi: 10.4103/0976-7800.109633

Marvibaigi, M., Supriyanto, E., Amini, N., Majid, F. A. A., & Jaganathan, S. K. (2014). Preclinical and clinical effects of mistletoe against breast cancer. *BioMed Research International, Volume 2014,* article ID 785479. doi: 10.1155/2014/785479

Mehasseb, M. K. & Habiba, M. A. (2009). Adenomyosis uteri: An update. *The Obstetrician and Gynaecologist, 11,* 41-47. doi: 10.1576/toag.11.1.41.27467

Meredith, S. M., Sanchez-Ramos, L., & Kaunitz, A. M. (2009). Diagnostic accuracy of transvaginal sonography for the diagnosis of adenomyosis: Systematic review and meta-analysis. *American Journal of Obstetrics and Gynecology, 201:107.*e1-6. doi: 10.1016/j.ajog.2009.03.021

Millischer, A., Borghese, B., Santulli, P., Lecomte, M., Dousset, B., & Chapron, C. (2013). Could adenomyosis be considered as a marker of severity in intestinal endometriosis? *Ultrasound in Obstetrics and Gynecology, 42:4.* doi: 10.1002/uog.12590

Missmer, S. A., Chavarro, J. E., Malspeis, S., Bertone-Johnson, E. R., & Hornstein, M. D. (2010). A prospective study of dietary fat consumption and endometriosis risk. *Human Reproduction, 25(6),* 1528-35. doi: 10.1093/humrep/deq044

Molinas, C. R., & Campo, R. (2006). Office hysteroscopy and adenomyosis. *Best Practice and Research Clinical Obstetrics and Gynaecology, 20(4),* 557-67. Retrieved from http://www.ncbi.nlm.nih.gov/pubmed/16554185

Moore, R. W., Rudy, T. A., Lin, T. M., Ko, K., & Peterson, R. E. (2001).

Abnormalities of sexual development in male rats with in utero and lactational exposure to the antiandrogenic plasticizer di(2-ethylhexyl) phthalate. *Environmental Health Perspectives, 109(3),* 229-237. Retrieved from http://www.ncbi.nlm.nih.gov/pmc/articles/PMC 1240240

National Institutes of Health. (2016). Black cohosh. Retrieved from https://ods.od.nih.gov/factsheets/BlackCohosh-HealthProfessional/

Noda, Y., Matsumoto, H., Umaoka, Y., Tatsumi, K., Kishi, J., & Mori, T. (1991). Involvement of superoxide radicals in the mouse two-cell block. *Molecular Reproduction and Development, 28(4),* 356-60. Retrieved from http://www.ncbi.nlm.nih.gov/pubmed/1648368

Northrup, C. (2016). Estrogen Dominance. Retrieved from http://www.drnorthrup.com/estrogen-dominance/

Novellas, S., Chassang, M., Delotte, J., Toullalan, O., Chevallier, A., Boouasis, J., & Chevallier, P. (2011). MRI characteristics of the uterine junctional zone: From normal to the diagnosis of adenomyosis. *American Journal of Roentgenology, 196(5).* doi: 10.2214/AJR.10.4877

Ochoa-Maya, M. R. (2012). Treatment considerations for excess estrogen and estrogen dominance. *Freedom to Heal.* Retrieved from http://www.freedomtoheal.org/2012/08/treatment-considerations-for-excess.html

Oh, S. J., Shin, J. H., Kim, T. H., Lee, H. S., Yoo, J. Y., Ahn, J. Y.,…Jeong, J. W. (2013). B-catenin activation contributes to the pathogenesis of adenomyosis through epithelial-mesenchymal transition. *Journal of Pathology, 231(2),* 210-222. doi: 10.1002/path.4224

Osada, H., Silberb, S., Kakinuma, T., Nagaishia, M., Katoc, K., & Katoc, O. (2010). Surgical procedure to conserve the uterus for future pregnancy in patients suffering from massive adenomyosis. *Reproductive BioMedicine Online.* Retrieved from http://www.infertile.com/inthenew/sci/2010-09-RBMO-adenomyosis.htm

Ota, H., Igarashi, S., Hatazawa, J., & Tanaka, T. (1998). Is adenomyosis an immune disease? *Human Reproduction Update, 4(4),* 360-7. Retrieved from http://www.ncbi.nlm.nih.gov/pubmed/9825851

Overk, C. R., Yao, P., Chadwick, L. R., Nikolic, D., Sun, Y., Cuendet, M. A.,…Bolton, J. L. (2005). Comparison of the in vitro estrogenic activities of compounds from hops (humulus lupulus) and red clover (trifolium pratense). *Journal of Agriculture and Food Chemistry, 53(16),* 6246-53. Retrieved from http://ncbi.nlm.nih.gov/pubmed/16076101

Owalbi, T. O., & Strickler, R. C. (1977). Adenomyosis: A neglected diagnosis. *Obstetrics and Gynecology, 50(4),* 424-7. Retrieved from www.ncbi.nlm.nih.gov/pubmed/904805

Pagedas, A. C., Bae, I. H., & Perkins, H. E. (1995). Review of 24 cases of uterine ablation failure. *Journal of Minimally Invasive Gynecology, 2(4),* S39. doi: http://dx.doi.org/10.1016/S1074-3804(05)80588-2

Panganamamula, U. R., Harmanli, O. H., Isik-Akbay, E. F., Grotegut, C. A., Dandolu, V., & Gaughan, J. P. (2004) Is prior uterine surgery a risk factor for adenomyosis? *Obstetrics and Gynecology, 104(5),* 1034-1038. doi:10.1097/01.AOG.0000143264.59822.73

Parazzini, F., Vercellini, P., Panazza, S., Chatenoud, L., Oldani, S., & Crosignani, P. (1997) Risk factors for adenomyosis. *Human Reproduction, 12(6),* 1275-1279. Retrieved from http://www.humrep.oxfordjournals.org/Content/12/6/1275.full.pdf

Parazzini, F., Paola, V., Candiani, M., & Fedele, L. (2013). Diet and endometriosis risk: A literature review. *Reproductive Biomedicine Online, 26(4), 323-336.* doi: 10.1016/j.rbmo.2012.12.011

Patisaul, H. & Jefferson, W. (2010). The pros and cons of phytoestrogens. *Frontiers in Neuroendocrinology, 31(4),* 400-419. doi: 10.1016/i.vfrne.2010.03.003

Peat, R. (2014). Progesterone, pregnenolone & DHEA – Three youth-associated hormones. Retrieved from http://raypeat.com/articles/articles/three-hormones.shtml

Powers, C. N. & Setzer, W. N. (2015). A molecular docking study of phytochemical estrogen mimics from dietary herbal supplements. *In Silico Pharmacology, 3,* 4. doi: 10.1186/s40203-015-0008-z

Rato, A. G., Pedrero, J. G., Martinez, M. A., Rio, B. D., Lazo, P. D., & Ramos, S. (1999). Melatonin blocks the activation of estrogen receptor for DNA binding. *FASEB Journal, 13(8),* 857-868. Retrieved from http://www.fasebj.org/content/13/8/857.full

Rebbeck, T. R., Troxel, A. B., Norman, S., Bunin, G. R., DeMichele, A., Baumgarten, M.,...Strom, B. L. (2007). A retrospective case-control study of the use of hormone-related supplements and association with breast cancer. *International Journal of Cancer, 120,* 1523-1528. doi:10.1002/ijc.22485

Reinhold, C., McCarthy, S., Bret, P. M., Mehio, A., Atri, M., Zakarian, R.,... Seymour, R. J. (1996) Diffuse adenomyosis: Comparison of endovaginal US and MR imaging with histopathologic correlation. *Radiology, 199(1),* 151-8. Retrieved from http://www.ncbi.nlm.nih.gov/pubmed/8633139

Rocha, A. L. L., Reis, F., & Taylor, R. (2013). Angiogenesis and endometriosis. *Obstetrics and Gynecology International, 2013,* Article ID 859619. doi: 10.1155/2013/859619

Rudin, D. & Felix, C. (1996). Omega-3 Oils, A Practical Guide. US: Avery.

Safirstein, A. (2015). Estrogen Dominance. Retrieved from http://fromcancertohealth.com/estrogen-dominance/

Schliep, K. C., Schisterman, E. F., Mumford, S. L., Pollack, A. Z., Zhang, C., Ye, A.,...Wactawski-Wende, J. (2012) Caffeinated beverage intake and reproductive hormones among premenopausal women in the biocycle study. *The American Journal of Clinical Nutrition, 95(2),* 488-497. doi: 10.3945/acjn.111.021287

Schlumpf, M., Durrer, S., Faass, O., Ehnes, C., Fuetsch, M., Gaille, C.,... Lichtensteiger, W. (2008). Developmental toxicity of UV filters and environmental exposure: A review. *International Journal of Andrology, 31(2),* 144-51. doi:10.1111/j.1365-2605.2007.00856.x

Seidl, M. M. & Stewart, D. C. (1998). Alternative treatments for menopausal symptoms: Systematic review of scientific and lay literature. *Canadian Family Physician, volume 44.* Retrieved from http://www.europepmc.org/backend/ptpmcrender.fcgi?accid=PMC2278270&blobtype=pdf

Sengupta, P., Sharma, A., Mazumdar, G., Banerjee, I., Tripathi, S., Bagchi, C., & Das, N. (2013). The possible role of fluoxetine in adenomyosis: An animal experiment with clinical correlations. *Journal of Clinical and Diagnostic Research, 7(7),* 1530-1534. doi: 10.7860/JCDR/2013/5654.3128

Sheng, J., Zhang, W. Y., Zhang, J. P., & Lu, D. (2009). The LNS-IUS study on adenomyosis: A 3-year follow-up study on the efficacy and side effects of the use of levonorgestrol intrauterine system for the treatment of dysmenorrhea associated with adenomyosis. *Contraception, 79(3),* 189-93. doi: 10.1016/j.contraception.2008.11.004

Shrestha, A. & Sedai, L. B. (2012). Understanding clinical features of adenomyosis: A case control study. *Nepal Medical College Journal, 14(3),* 176-9. Retrieved from http://www.ncbi.nlm.nih.gov/pubmed/24047010

Siskin, G. P., Tublin, M. E., Stainken, B. F., Dowling, K., & Dolen, E. G. (2001). Uterine artery embolization for the treatment of adenomyosis: Clinical response and evaluation with MR imaging. *American Journal of Roentgenology, 177(2),* 297-302. Retrieved from http://www.ncbi.nlm.nih.gov/pubmed/11461849

Slomczynska, M. (2008). Xenoestrogens: Mechanisms of action and some detection studies. *Polish Journal of Veterinary Sciences, 11(3),* 263-9. Retrieved from http://www.ncbi.nlm.nih.gov/pubmed/18942551

Smith, Elizabeth (2004). Adenomyosis. Retrieved from http://www.adeno101.com/

Smith, Elizabeth (2014). How to avoid xenoestrogens that cause adenomyosis. Retrieved from http://www.adeno101.com/xeno.htm

Soysal, S., Soysal, M. E., Ozer, S., Gul, N., & Gezgin, T. (2004). The effects of post-surgical administration of goserelin plus anastrozole compared to goserelin alone in patients with severe endometriosis: A prospective randomized trial. *Human Reproduction, 19(1),* 160. doi: 10.1093/humanrep/deh035

Streuli, I., Dubuisson, J., Santulli, P., de Ziegler, D., Batteux, F., & Chapron, C. (2014). An update on the pharmacological management of adenomyosis. *Expert Opinion on Pharmacotherapy, 15(16),* 2347-2360. doi: 10.1517/14656566.2014.953055

Tao, J., Zhang, P., Liu, G., Yan, H., Bu, X., Ma, Z.,...Jia, W. (2009). Cytotoxicity of Chinese motherwort (yimucao) aqueous ethanol extract is non-apoptotic and estrogen receptor independent on human breast cancer cells. *Journal of Ethnopharmacology, 122(2),* 234-9. Retrieved fromhttp://www.ncbi.nlm.nih.gov/pubmed/19330917

Taran, F. A., Weaver, A. L., Coddington, C. C., & Stewart, E. A. (2010). Understanding adenomyosis: A case control study. *Fertility and Sterility, 94(4),* 1223-8. doi: 10.1016/j.fertnstert.2009.06.049

Taran, F. A., Stewart, E. A., & Brucker, S. (2013). Adenomyosis:

Epidemiology, risk factors, clinical phenotype and surgical and interventional alternatives to hysterectomy. *Geburtshilfe Frauenheilkd, 73(9),* 924-931. doi: 10.1055/s-0033-1350840

Taylor, H. S. (2000). The role of HOX genes in human implantation. *Human Reproduction Update, 6(1),* 75-9. Retrieved from http://www.ncbi.nlm.nih.gov/pubmed/10711832

The Dr. Oz Show. (2015). Soy: The good, the bad and the best. Retrieved from http://www.doctoroz.com/print/45041

Thompson, J. F. (2016). Exam 5 Review: Chapter 27 Uterine Anatomy. In *Austin Peay State University Biology Website.* Retrieved from www.apsubiology.org/anatomy/2020/2020_Exam_Reviews/Exam_s/CH27_Uterine_Anatomy.htm

Tokyol, C., Aktepe, F., Dilek, F. H., Sahin, O., & Arioz, D. T. (2009). Expression of cyclooxygenase-2 and matrix metalloproteinase-2 in adenomyosis and endometrial polyps and its correlation with angiogenesis. *International Journal of Gynecological Pathology, 28(2),* 148-56. doi: 10.1097/ PGP.0b013e318187033b

Tomio, K., Kawana, K., Taguchi, A., Isobe, Y., Iwamoto, R., Yamashita, A.,...Kojima, S. (2013). Omega-3 polyunsaturated fatty acids suppress the cystic lesion formation of peritoneal endometriosis in transgenic mouse models. *PLoS ONE, 8(9),* e73085. doi: 10.1371/journal/pone.0073085

University of Maryland Medical Center. (2016). Evening primrose oil (EPO). In *Complementary and Alternative Medicine Guide – Herbs.* Retrieved from http://www.umm.edu/health/medical/altmed/herb/evening-primrose-oil

Upson, K., DeRoos, A. J., Thompson, M. L., Sathyanarayana, S., Scholes, D., Barr, D. B., & Holt, V. L. Organochlorine pesticides and risk of endometriosis: Findings from a population-based case-control study. (2013) *Environmental Health Perspectives, 121,* 11-12. doi: 10.1289/ehp.1306648

van der Woude, H., Ter Veld, M. G., Jacobs, N., van der Saag, P. T., Murk, A. J., & Rietjens, I. M. (2005). The stimulation of cell proliferation by quercetin is mediated by the estrogen receptor. *Molecular Nutrition and Food Research, 49(8),* 763-71. Retrieved from http://www.ncbi.nlm.nih.gov/pubmed/15937998

Vercellini, P., Consonni, D., Dridi, D., Bracco, B., Frattaruolo, M. P., &

Somigliana, E. (2014). Uterine adenomyosis and in vitro fertilization outcome: A systematic review and meta-analysis. *Human Reproduction, 29:5,* 964-77. Retrieved from http://www.unboundmedicine.com/medline/citation/24622619/Uterine_adenomyosis_and_in_vitro_fertilization_outcome:a_systematic_review_and_meta_analysis

Wang, J., Zhang, H. H., &Duan, H. (2010). Expression of ERα in endometrial-myometrial interface of human adenomyosis. *Zhonghua Yi Xue Za Zhi, 90(27),* 1914-17. Retrieved from http://www.ncbi.nlm.nih.gov/pubmed/20979911

WebMD.com (2016). Anise. In *Vitamins and Supplements.* Retrieved from http://www.webmd.com/vitamins-supplements/ingredientmono-582-anise.aspx?activeingredientid=582&activeingredientname=anise

WebMD.com (2016). Indole-3-carbinol. In *Vitamins and Supplements.* Retrieved from http://www.webmd.com/vitamins-supplements/ingredientmono-1027-indole-3-carbinol.aspx?activeingredientid=1027&

WebMD.com (2016). Licorice. In *Vitamins and Supplements.* Retrieved from http://www.webmd.com/vitamins-supplements/indredientmono-881-LICORICE.aspx?activeIngredientId=881&activeIngredientName=LICORICE

WebMD.com (2016). Pyridoxine (vitamin B6). In *Vitamins and Supplements.* Retrieved from www.webmd.com/vitamins-supplements/ingredientmono-934-pyridoxine%20vitamin%20b6.aspx?activeingredientid=934&

WebMD.com (2016). Thyme. In *Vitamins and Supplements.* Retrieved from http://www.webmd.com/vitamins-supplements/ingredientmono-823-thyme.aspx?activeingredient=823&activeingredientname=thyme

WebMD.com (2016). Turmeric. In *Vitamins and Supplements.* Retrieved from http://www.webmd.com/vitamins-supplements/ingredientmono-662-turmeric.aspx?activeingredientid=662

Weil, A. (2000). Eating Well for Optimum Health. New York: Alfred A. Knopf

WholeHealthMD.com (2005). Chasteberry. In *Supplements.* Retrieved from http:// www.wholehealthmd.com/ME2/dirmod.asp?type=AWHN_Supplements&tier=2&id=B876FF3FB5FE45E7AC1B9AB8D2E94726

WholeHealthMD.com (2005). False unicorn root. In *Supplements.* Retrieved from http://www.wholehealthmd.com/ME2/dirmod.asp?nm= Reference+Library&type=AWHN_Suplenents&mod=Supplements& tier=2&id=7E1C4F44E54C42CEB

Wortman, M. & Daggett, A. (2001). Reoperative hysteroscopic surgery in the management of patients who fail endometrial ablation and resection. *Journal of the American Association of Gynecologic Laparoscopists, 8(2),* 272-7. Retrieved from www.ncbi.nlm.nih.gov/pubmed/11342737

Yamanaka, A., Kimura, F., Kishi, Y., Takahashi, K., Suginami, H., Shimizu, Y., & Murakami, T. (2014). Progesterone and synthetic progestin, dienogest, induce apoptosis of human primary cultures of adenomyotic stromal cells. *European Journal of Obstetrics & Gynecology and Reproductive Biology, 179,* 170-4. doi: 10.1016/j.ejogrb.2014.05.031

Yeager, M. (2012). My Hormones Are Killing Me: Living with Adenomyosis and Estrogen Dominance. U.S.: Maria Yeager

Yeager, M. (2012). The Health Benefits of Omega-3 Fatty Acids in Inflammatory Bowel Disease and Irritable Bowel Syndrome. U.S.: Maria Yeager

Yen, C. F., Basar, M., Kizilay, G., Lee, C. L., Kayisli, U. A., & Arici, A. (2006) Implantation markers are decreased in endometrium of women with adenomyosis during the implantation window. *Fertility and Sterility, 86(3),* S338. doi: http://dx.doi.org/10.1016/j.fertnstert.2006.07.919

Zava, D. T., Dollbaum, C. M., & Blen, M. (1998). Estrogen and progestin bioactivity of foods, herbs, and spices. *The Proceedings of the Society for Experimental Biology and Medicine, 7(3),* 369-78. Retrieved from http://www.cancersupportivecare.com/estrogenherb.html

Zhi, X., Honda, K., Ozaki, K., Misugi, T., Sumi, T., & Ishiko, O. (2007). Dandelion T-1 extract up-regulates reproductive hormone receptor expression in mice. *International Journal of Molecular Medicine, 20(3),* 287-92. Retrieved from http://www.ncbi.nlm.nih.gov/pubmed/17671731

Printed in Great Britain
by Amazon